Bob Brody's remarkable true-life stories offer hope to those who need it most: people who are surviving cancer. We admire athletes for their physical prowess on the field; *Edge Against Cancer* introduces us to several athletes who are heroes in recovery, too. From Mario Lemieux to Fred Lebow, *Edge Against Cancer* presents an all-star team of courage in the face of cancer. Bob Brody even provides some surprising scientific evidence that the "jock factor" could be a path that others can follow to survive cancer. Confronted with an athlete's focus and competitive spirit, cancer could be considered an opponent waiting for defeat.

—Dan Rather
CBS News

EDGE
AGAINST
CANCER

By Robert Brody

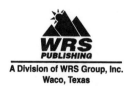

WRS
PUBLISHING
A Division of WRS Group, Inc.
Waco, Texas

First published in the United States of America in 1993 by WRS Publishing, A Division of WRS Group, Inc., 701 N. New Road, Waco, Texas 76710
Book design by Kenneth Turbeville
Jacket design by Talmage Minter and Joe James
Back jacket photo credit: Norman Collection
Back jacket photo credit: Griffith Collection
Back jacket photo credit: Norman Collection
Back jacket photo credit: Lebow Collection

10 9 8 7 6 5 4 3 2 1

Library of Congress Cataloging in Publication Data

Brody, Robert (Robert Leon), 1952 -
      Edge against cancer / by Robert Brody.
            p.   cm.
      ISBN 1-56796-016-2 : $12.95
      1. Cancer--Psychological aspects.   2. Athletes--Health.
      3. Athletes--Psychology.   I. Title.
      RC262.B76   1993
      616.99'4'0019--dc20
                                                                        93-30554
                                                                        CIP

For Elvira

Table Of Contents

Foreword

I've practiced sports medicine long enough to know that elite athletes, with rare exceptions, deal better with physical adversity than the rest of us. For proof, we need look no further than Bo Jackson, the White Sox outfielder and former NFL running back who, despite a severely dislocated hip, has rehabilitated himself back into the lineup. I believe such comebacks have little to do with physiology—or, for that matter, the gifts of genetic endowment—and everything to do with attitude.

Example: Earvin "Magic" Johnson, told he was HIV-positive, could have crawled into a shell. Instead, the peerless Los Angeles Lakers point guard directly confronted his fears, went public, and stepped forward as an advocate for AIDS awareness. He also cleared away enough time to excel in the 1992 Barcelona Olympics. In all my years as a physician, I've witnessed countless such examples of this singularly vital dimension in the athletic makeup: mental resilience.

I've seen athletes struck down by every injury imaginable, facing the most dire diagnoses and the dimmest prospects of a comeback, only to pull themselves back together and get out there to compete again. The answer: attitude. Every athlete who excels—indeed, every executive, every ditch-digger, every housewife—has a special mindset that yields successful performance. Why, then, would this attitude not apply to cancer as well? Like injury, cancer is a physical setback one can cope with if blessed with the will, the resourcefulness, the toughness, and the tenacity.

This book reveals a truth I have long believed: that top athletes have an advantage over most of us—an edge, as the title of this book indicates—that is tempered, as if by a blacksmith, in the heat of competition; and that, moreover, this attitude is an invaluable asset in dealing not only with a sprained rotator cuff but also the crucible of a disease as severe as cancer. I agree with the author: equipped with this attitude, we, too, can learn to survive anything.

—Lyle J. Micheli, M.D.
Past President, American College of Sports Medicine
Harvard Medical School Professor

Introduction

This book started as a whisper of an idea. I had heard in recent years about one athlete after another who had survived cancer and come back to compete again in sports. These athletes seemed to have taken up the gauntlet and gone from diagnosis and treatment to recovery and rehabilitation with remarkable success. I sensed the presence of certain telltale similarities—common denominators—among the athletes, most notably simple survival strategies. What, if anything, might this pattern signify?

The images of these highly successful athletes trading the team uniform for the hospital gown and coming through with career and identity intact aroused questions never before posed. Do athletes, especially those of elite caliber, possess an advantage over the average person in coping with and recovering from this ever-present, multifaceted disease we call cancer? Are superior athletes who specialize in superior physical performance, and routinely endure pain, fatigue and injury, better equipped for the challenge of this disease, more likely to have higher cure rates, by virtue of certain emotional qualities, than you or I? Might athletes respond to the adversities of cancer not only because they are more fleet of foot, more nimble, more powerful than we, but also because they bring to bear singular powers of focus and competitive drive in such a confrontation?

Maybe so.

Then again, maybe not.

On reflection, the idea seemed off the wall. After all, every year cancer strikes about 1.5 million Americans, nearly half of whom die as a direct result. The disease is a matter of cells gone amok, regardless of your occupation. Period. These renegade cells multiply and destroy the body, whether the patient is an Olympic sprinter or the most sedentary slob. Case closed. End of story.

Still, the whisper grew insistent. So I performed what you might call exploratory surgery. I asked around, questioning cancer specialists and sports psychologists. And I received encouraging answers—to wit, the experts pronounced my questions serious and scientifically valid. With that as my backstop, I formed a theory that athletes may be endowed with a unique attitude— here dubbed the Jock Factor—that can combat cancer.

I felt certain from the outset that although I could track down all kinds of data on cancer causes and epidemiology, nothing would more vividly reveal this hypothesis, with all its respective merits and flaws, than accounts of athletes who had survived cancer and returned to compete anew. So here are profiles of eight athletes—a cross-section of men and women, young and middle-aged, professional and amateur, from hither and yon around the United States—plus a Greek chorus of family members, friends, teammates, coaches, and physicians. These eight athletes span the spectrum of sports from baseball, football, and soccer to golf, skiing, wrestling, marathon running, hockey, triathlons, and arm wrestling. They are currently in remission from an array of cancers, including tumors of the brain, bone, breast, skin, testicles, ovaries, and lymphatic system.

Only in the last chapter do I come to conclusions. The final pages bring together the latest research, including a survey of American College of Sports Medicine members commissioned exclusively for this book, as well as expert opinion from notable medical specialists. About 1,500 Americans will die of cancer *every day* this year. Obviously, we need more research on the prevention, detection, and treatment of this scourge. What we need even more is the hope that we and those we love can survive cancer. I believe that the stories of these eight athletes may yield clues to, and even impart valuable lessons about, such survival—and take a small step toward inspiring such hope. After all, even a whisper can echo into the future.

Chapter 1

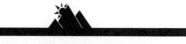

JEFF BANISTER:
TWICE BLESSED

If you live in LaMarque, Texas, your father probably busts his butt in a petroleum plant. The town of 16,000, sprawling along Galveston Bay near the Gulf of Mexico, is all about oil. Vast dripping tankers steam into port bearing the precious cargo. Roughnecks work the rigs, and the folks in the refineries go home in need of a second pass at some industrial soap. Through it all, the oil comes and goes in an ebb and flow of import-export.

Until about 1970, the railroad tracks that cut through LaMarque divided the blacks from the whites. LaMarque High School, positioned on one side, stayed all white, while Lincoln High School, on the other, stayed black. You kept to your own side of the tracks unless you were bucking for trouble. The same unspoken rule applied to the local football games: all the whites in the stands here, all the blacks there. Some small towns in Texas just came around late in the game to racial integration.

Back in 1969, Bob Banister coached the LaMarque High School football team, and his boys played hard, industrial-strength, Texas football. That's because the team followed his orders, and because blue-collar towns put more stock in force than in finesse. Bob, a former college football player who hailed from Oklahoma, stood 6 feet, 3 inches and weighed 230 pounds. He looked like a rugged customer, so players obeyed him. On many a Friday night, just about everyone in LaMarque gathered at the high school field for football, the preferred family entertainment in town, with Bob Banister at the helm of it all. As the saying goes, Texas has only two sports—football and spring football.

Jeff Banister liked baseball better, and that was okay with Bob, his father. In LaMarque, baseball took a back seat to football, but not by much. The town had plenty of sandlots and corner parks carved out for baseball. Baseball was a central activity there, especially in the summer. Jeff started playing at the age of 5, when his father bought him a glove and a ball and played catch with him. The boy wanted to go to a two-week summer baseball camp, even though all the other kids there were 7 or 8 and much larger. His father pulled strings with the high school baseball coach, who ran the camp, to get him inside the gates.

The next spring, when Jeff was in first grade, the local elementary school held Little League tryouts. The blond-haired, blue-eyed boy went home and asked his father if he could sign up, and the answer was yes, of course, go ahead. Jeff was shorter and lighter than the other boys, his jeans usually drooping off his behind, but Jeff tried out and made the team. Jeff liked to play baseball and he excelled. In pickup games, he was always one of the first kids chosen.

Jeff had a slingshot arm and he could hit the ball, and even if he was hardly the most graceful fielder, two out of three skills would do for the time being. Mainly, Jeff could whack the ball, and far, too. He smacked his first Little League home run, right over the fence, at the age of 8. He liked to take his cuts at the plate, because that gave you your turn in the spotlight, just you and the pitcher going one-on-one, eyeball to eyeball. And no sport had a better feeling than that of laying good wood on the ball. Nothing else even came close, because hitting a baseball is the most difficult act in all of sports—there's so little time to see the ball sail in, so little opportunity to whip the bat around and hope to connect squarely. But Jeff could do it. He could bop the ball right over the fence.

Little League games in LaMarque took place at a local landmark, Bobby Beach Stadium. Young Bobby Beach was beaned with a pitch in the mid-1960s and had gone to the hospital and died. His father, owner of the Beach Construction Company, decided to build a memorial and name the place after his beloved son. That's how Bobby Beach Stadium came to be. It was splendid, too, like nothing else in LaMarque, like nothing else for miles around. The covered grandstand wrapped around the diamond, from first base to third, and if all the seats filled up—as often happened—folks brought lawn chairs from home to set right on the field. The town manicured the grass as if tending to a PGA putting green. All along the outfield fences were advertisements for oil companies and credit unions and maybe a savings and loan or two. Floodlights for night contests bathed the field in a facsimile of sunshine. Those lights beamed so brightly that, from the next town over, you would know for certain where everyone in LaMarque had gone for the night.

Jeff graduated to the larger field at Bobby Beach Stadium when he was 9 years old. He promptly dispatched a pitch over the centerfield fence, quite a shot—270 feet and change—for a skinny kid like him. That inaugural blast was a grand slam, too, and brought Jeff a degree of small-town celebrity. The local bank president sent him a congratulatory letter along with a set of new, shiny American coins, all encased in hard plastic. Jeff hit six home runs his first year on the big field and 10 the next, both times leading his team, the Integrity Incorporated Eagles (sponsored by a firm of local private investigators). As he passed through LaMarque, folks would say, "That's Jeff Banister. Good baseball player."

Bob Banister taught his son that the point was to go out there and have some fun. Sure, the man wanted to win games. But if he had learned anything as a coach over the years, it was that before you can succeed you have to fail, and so you might as well get a kick out of the game. Bob never barked at Jeff from the sidelines that he should do this and do that. Not at all. He had borne witness to many a father bellowing from behind the batting cage that his adolescent son should plant his feet like this, get his elbows out like that. Fools. The technique would come. Meanwhile, he would just let Jeff play, let him learn on his own, more or less, and at his own pace. The key was to have fun.

Jeff either went to class or played baseball, nothing in between. He watched few baseball games on television, because all the fun was in the doing. He preferred the sandlot pick-up games to Little League, with its universe of parents and uniforms and official scorekeepers. On the sandlot, you had no coaches or crowds distracting you. It was just you and your buddies choosing up sides and playing the game. You played all day and nobody made you stop after seven innings, and your parents never questioned your whereabouts because they knew where you were and what you were doing. You were out there playing over at the field in the park behind the houses across the street, squeezing in a few innings even if only four boys showed up. And if it rained, you all got together on a patio or in a garage, and you hit rocks with a stick or whatever implement was handy. That was the deal: baseball anytime, anywhere, with anyone.

❦ ❦ ❦

When Jeff turned 12, a Little League coach asked Bob Banister for permission to play his son as catcher. His father said if it was okay with the boy, it was okay with him. It turned out that Jeff, until then either a shortstop or an outfielder, liked the idea. Why not? he thought.

From the first game on, Jeff knew he was meant to play catcher. The position had so much going for it. You hunkered down behind the batter, wearing a mask and chest protector and shinguards, and flicked signals to the pitcher. You were smack in the thick of the action, the quarterback on the baseball field. You saw the whole game and were involved with every decision, every pitch. You felt responsible, because it took some brains to call the shots.

But most of all Jeff liked getting dirty. He liked getting hot and sweaty down there in the dirt behind the plate. He could get as dirty and sweaty as the roughnecks who worked the oil rigs all over LaMarque. He never had to care how he looked, unlike the pitcher, who always wanted to keep his uniform clean in the limelight. Catching was more physical than any other position except pitcher, and Jeff liked the hurly-burly of it. Your knees and feet and back might hurt because it was taxing as all get-out, but after a game, you felt you had accomplished something important and dropped into sleep as if leaping off a cliff. The fans might think you were hardly working, that you just squatted there, caught the ball, tossed it back to the mound. But your teammates and coaches appreciated what went into catching, and none more so than the pitcher. If the pitcher trusted your instincts and had confidence in you, the whole team would.

By the end of that first summer as a catcher, the change in position had brought out Jeff's competitive instincts as nothing else ever had. If an opponent tried to mow Jeff down in the base path for a run, he always blocked the plate. As a batter, he always hankered to face the best pitcher. If he felt he had played poorly, he would fault himself. If his team lost, he got upset. Jeff kept bashing home runs, and folks in LaMarque went over to him after games to tell him he was good, and success begot success. The better he performed, the more he wanted to improve.

But however competitive he became, Jeff always remembered that his father was boss. Bob Banister could let the boy know what he wanted him to know without coming right out and saying it. He had his rules and you were going to play by those rules. If he told you to be home at ten o'clock, you had better be in at ten o'clock, and if he had to, he would give you a good smart smack on the behind. But usually Bob kept his hands to himself because he was 6 feet, 3 inches and 230 pounds, and for him to lay a finger on Jeff was redundant. All the coach had to do to straighten out his 12-year-old, really, was just to stand there. He would loom over him and block out the sun and look him in the eye, and Jeff would feel engulfed by a shadow of irrefutable authority. The boy would think, Well, whatever my Dad wants done I'd better do, and quick.

As a teenager, Jeff gave him a run for his money. He had ideas of his own that he felt no hesitation about expressing. Sometimes his mother, Verda, a high school teacher, would feel like pulling out her hair. One time Jeff was hanging around with some friends who decided, just as a lark, to rip a pay telephone off a wall, and that made him a sort of accomplice. On another occasion, Jeff and a friend took some two-by-fours out of shop class and slipped the boards through the door handles at both ends of a corridor in junior high school. That locked the doors. When the school bell rang, students trying to get to class found themselves imprisoned in the hallway for 15 minutes. The principal forced the perpetrators to stay after school for a week to clean the bathrooms. Jeff begged him to guard the news from his father. The principal, knowing Bob Banister to be a merciless disciplinarian, kept quiet.

But never, in all those years of living at home, did Jeff ever feel that his father took him to task unfairly. If he got into trouble, he knew he had it coming to him, knew his father just wanted him to do right.

As the boy got older, Bob came to expect more out of him, and told him so. He taught his son that once he started a job, he should finish it, no matter what. Jeff knew that abiding by this credo would make life more difficult for him, but if he ever felt like quitting anything, he would remember what his father had advised and stick it out.

When he joined the junior teenage league at LaMarque High School, Jeff was only 5 feet, 6 inches and 135 pounds (after a shower), with long arms and no excess of muscle. In appearance—not in spirit—he made an unlikely catcher. Typically, the guy behind the plate is a hulk, a human backstop. And here was Banister, narrow of frame, challenging opponents coming down the third base line to steamroll right over him. And many a time that's exactly what happened. Sometimes, while being run over, Jeff would tag out the base runner, but he himself would always get the worst of it. Those plays would leave his elbows and knees all scratched up, his chin gashed, or his nose bleeding.

In high school Jeff first formed the clear-eyed ambition to be a major-league baseball player. In the late 1970s, professional catchers were more widely recognized than ever as all-around, highly paid players. Johnny Bench, Carlton Fisk, Gary Carter, and Bob Boone had made the difference. All Jeff could think about—whether sitting in chemistry class or eating dinner with his family—was playing catcher in the pros.

He would fantasize about stepping to the plate in the pros with the bases juiced and the score locked, the crowd going nuts and the announcer, breathless, shouting that here came Jeff Banister, always a threat to hammer the big blow and win the game. In this daydream, Jeff always imagined himself confronting the pitcher, eyeball to eyeball. Like most 16-year-olds, Jeff felt healthy and strong, felt he could run through walls. He felt immortal. He would never get tired, never get hurt. And he would certainly never come close to dying.

He was mistaken.

❦ ❦ ❦

In November 1982, Jeff was playing a football game, a quarter final in the state playoffs, in the Houston Astrodome. He'd joined the high school football team as a linebacker, if only to keep himself in shape for baseball season. During one play in the game, Jeff collided with a blocker on the opposing team and rose from the pile with a twisted left ankle. Right away the ankle swelled, but despite the pain he stayed in the game. He had never during his whole football career come out of a game because of injury.

Afterward, the twisted ankle continued to bring him severe pain. He tried to stop thinking about it, hoped it would go away of its own accord. But for some reason, it failed to heal. He listened to advice from the team trainer and applied ice, but the ankle kept aching and throbbing, so much so that Jeff developed a limp and quit all sports. He would wake in the morning, get out of bed to take a step, and the soreness in his ankle would startle him. One Saturday night, Jeff was supposed to go to a dance with a date, but when the girl arrived, his ankle hurt so severely they stayed at his house.

On Monday, January 15, 1983, his 17th birthday, Jeff stayed home from school, and his mother drove him to see Dr. Leroy Lockhardt, a gray-haired family practitioner. After taking X-rays and injecting Jeff with penicillin shots, Dr. Lockhardt recommended that Jeff go home and wrap the ankle.

The next day, still in serious pain, Jeff stayed home from school again. His ankle ballooned to the size of a grapefruit. Alarmed at the sight—and unable to stand, much less walk—he crawled out of bed and slithered down the hallway on his elbows until he reached the phone. "I was in so much pain, I just wanted someone to come help me," Jeff recalled in his home-grown Texas twang. "I just wanted it to quit hurting and for someone to tell me what was wrong." He dialed the phone number of the junior high school where his mother taught mathematics and asked to speak with her. "Come home, Mom," he said. "My ankle is killing me." Verda Banister rushed home, only to find her boy passed out on his bedroom floor. She called her husband. When he arrived at the house, they carried Jeff to the car and drove him to the hospital.

A resident promptly wheeled the boy into the emergency room on a stretcher. His left ankle looked like a water balloon, all swollen with fluid and stretched tight, as if ready to explode. The physician on duty lightly tapped the bulging ankle with a scalpel. He accidentally lanced the injury right open. The skin splayed apart and pus spattered across the bed. Jeff howled and the doctor shot him with painkiller. Then the doctor realized he would need to take him in for emergency exploratory surgery, and knocked him out with general anesthesia.

During the surgery, Dr. Lockhardt found a cyst. He removed the growth from the ankle. Then he came out to tell the Banisters that the cyst suggested something worse.

"The doctors came into the recovery room and took my parents out into the hall," Jeff recalled. "I heard talking in the background as the doctors told my parents what was wrong. It seemed to be a big shock to everybody. My mom came back to my room and she was crying. My dad came over too, and they told me what was going on. I had a form of bone cancer. Something was eating at the bone in my leg. It was going to take some surgery to clear it up.

"I got scared. Real scared. I tried to be positive. But somewhere along the line I thought, I'm going to die. To me, the word 'cancer' meant death."

His father played it poker-faced. Jeff had seen him cry only twice, at the deaths of his father and his older sister. Now Bob Banister said, "Jeff, when you've gotten down, you've always come back on top. And that's what you're going to have to do now. Problems happen for a reason, and you've got to come out fighting."

"When I got cancer," Jeff said, "I think my father felt it would be easier on me if he refused to show me that it was tough on him. But he was always an optimist. The consensus for my parents and everyone involved was that we would have to fight it. My mother and father told me I would be all right, and that gave me hope. From that point on, I decided I was not going to let the cancer beat me." Jeff would hunker down in the dirt and try to call the pitches.

❦ ❦ ❦

With the cyst out, Jeff took antibiotics to ward off infection and chemotherapy as an extra precaution. As the swelling in the ankle shrank and the fever died down, he seemed to be getting better. But a week later he came down with the same set of symptoms; his temperature shot to 103 and his ankle started to puff out again. Dr. Lockhardt scheduled him for surgery to take another look inside and discovered that another cyst had materialized in place of the previous one. This cyst, too, was removed. But remaining behind was a speck that Dr. Lockhardt suspected had started the problem.

For the next two weeks, as before, Jeff recuperated adequately. The inflamed ankle narrowed to normal size, his body temperature stabilized, and the terrible pain disappeared. Then he got sick again, and the same events recurred in exactly the same sequence. Fever. Swelling. Pain. Surgery. Yet a third cyst had cropped up on the leg, only higher along the bone, closer to the calf. And so Dr. Lockhardt performed yet a third operation to remove the new cyst. But the puzzling and worrisome speck remained beyond reach.

So it went, as a pattern established itself. On each go-round, Dr. Lockhardt took out a cyst and believed Jeff to be in the clear. For about two weeks, Jeff would heal from the surgery, take his medicine, and look forward to getting out of the hospital. The doctors would declare themselves optimistic about his prospects for recovery. The ravaged tissue inside the leg would regenerate itself and slowly grow back. But then, like those tricky birthday candles you blow out only to see the wicks burst into flames again, another cyst would take shape just above the location of its predecessor. The fever would burn so hot that the nurses would pack his leg in ice. The cysts crept higher and higher along his leg, inching closer to his calf and then his knee, eating away at the bone from the inside.

No matter what means of attack the doctors tried—no matter which combination of chemo and antibiotics was administered or how much tissue surrounding the cyst was scraped away—the growth always came back, full-blown and dangerous. Dr. Lockhardt had difficulty pinpointing the genesis of the cysts—except for the presence of that stubbornly ineradicable speck.

As weeks turned into months, the boy felt his relief and hope turn to disappointment and dread, only to revert again. Four times now Dr. Lockhardt had gone in to uproot the nagging cyst, and four times a new, equally menacing nodule had emerged. For Jeff, life took on the rhythm of stop-and-go traffic. Green light, red light. Green light, red light. Meanwhile, he lay in the hospital bed, unable to stand or walk.

Now his left leg was wasting away, probably all because of some damn speck, Jeff thought. In each operation, Lockhardt had to slice off a sheath of flesh from the ankle and gouge out tissue from inside the leg to tweezer out the cyst. All this cutting and digging had left the ankle with a gaping hole—"humongous," Jeff called it—that refused to heal. "I had to lie there day in and day out and see my ankle taken apart," he said. "Everything—all the flesh—was gone. The cancer was eating the bone right away. I was afraid it would turn my leg into dust."

The surgeries had scraped the ankle clean, pulled out not only cyst and bone, but also surrounding tissue and tendons and nerves. His left leg was now held together precariously. "It looked like some animal had gone in there and actually taken a big bite out of my ankle."

With the wound so wide open, his hospital room had to be kept sterile. Family and friends worried about bringing into the room an infection that would invade his leg. Visitors wore face masks, gloves, and gowns. Jeff began to feel like a specimen in a laboratory.

❦ ❦ ❦

Malignant bone tumors are rare, accounting for only about one in every 500 cancer cases in the United States. The disease strikes children more than adults. In the 1960s, when the only treatment was surgery, approximately four in five eventually died of bone cancer. Today, with new treatment regimens and advanced surgical techniques, one-half to three-fourths of all bone cancer patients who undergo chemotherapy survive.

The typical symptom for the disease is a complaint about pain. This pain is unrelated to what the patient is doing at the time and intensifies at night. Some patients suffer the growth of a tangible mass. To an infrequent degree patients also complain of fever, weight loss, and general malaise. An X-ray can detect a lesion and reveal whether it is benign or malignant. A bone scan, magnetic resonance imaging, or computerized axial tomography can determine the extent to which a malignancy has spread, if at all.

The most prevalent bone malignancy is osteosarcoma, especially in children and young adults. Most of these tumors are located around the knee. Often surgery can remove sections of bone that contain the tumor and thereby salvage the limb in question. The surgeon can then insert either a bone graft from a cadaver or a metal prosthesis to replace the missing sections. Chemotherapy combinations have proven effective against osteosarcoma, before and after surgery. Treatments typically involve agents such as methotrexate, doxorubicin, cyclophosphamide, and cisplatin.

❦ ❦ ❦

Friends and teammates would visit Jeff in the hospital and talk baseball. They knew that chewing the fat about baseball might help get him through the day. So the boys whiled away the hours talking about diving catches and perfect pegs and tape-measure home runs. Then everyone would leave and Jeff would lie there alone in his bed.

Sometimes he would watch soap operas and talk shows, at least until his eyes glazed over with indifference, never a long wait. Or he watched baseball games on television. But spectating gave him no solace at all—he had never gone for it much. He stayed in his bed surrounded by strangers—doctors and nurses and orderlies—nobody he could talk to personally for more than a minute or two, and he had to occupy himself, had to direct his mind toward something rewarding. So he daydreamed about baseball. On days when he felt especially blue—he worried about the accumulating medical bills, more than his parents, both of whom were public-school teachers, could comfortably cover—he would remember the pickup contests in the sandlots and corner parks of LaMarque, the days on the baseball field that never seemed to end, and he would feel safe again and altogether happy.

He saw himself working out again, training for his return to the sport with wind sprints and dumbbells, whatever it took. He envisioned himself out on the field, crouched behind the pitcher and nailing a would-be base stealer with a 12-gauge peg to second. Or standing at the plate and delivering a towering shot into the ozone. These thoughts would bring a smile.

Then a fifth cyst appeared. This cyst was growing faster than the others had, and the doctors, duly alarmed, immediately prepped Jeff for exploratory surgery again. His temperature soared to 104 degrees and Dr. Lockhardt, concerned that a higher fever might edge Jeff into a coma, ordered the nurses to pack him in ice from head to toe to cool him off. This fifth operation, different from its predecessors, might call for an extreme measure.

"Jeff," Dr. Lockhardt said, "we're going to have to operate

again. And while we're in surgery, we're going to have to make a decision." He explained to Jeff and his parents that he had to probe inside the leg to find the origin of the cysts—most likely that nettlesome speck—and determine just how fast and how far the latest version was spreading. He added, "It's a possibility we'll need to amputate your leg below the knee."

As Jeff and his folks took in this news, a long silence hung in the air. Jeff remembered a girl from high school who had developed bone cancer. The doctors had amputated her afflicted leg at the hip. Jeff imagined himself returning to high school with his left leg missing, imagined hopping around on crutches with his left pant leg folded back under at the knee. It would mean life without baseball for him. It was unbearable to imagine. "All I remember is being scared to death," he said.

Dr. Lockhardt began to walk out of the room. But before he reached the door, Jeff called out to him.

"You're not taking my leg," Jeff said.

The doctor stopped and turned around. "It may be a question of saving your life," he said.

"I would rather die than lose my leg."

"I am going to save your life before I save your leg."

"I would rather die than not be able to run," Jeff said.

Dr. Lockhardt—feeling sorry for Jeff and unsure what else to say—just looked point-blank at the 17-year-old boy. The doctor, himself a former college football player, had operated under traumatic circumstances as an Air Force medic in Vietnam. Now he was past 50, with a leathery face and a flinty look in his eye, but he retained a kind and understanding bedside manner. Dr. Lockhardt glanced at Bob and Verda and decided they should take it from there.

"My father and mother and I had this big discussion," Jeff recalled. "It was more of a crying session than anything. All of us were crying. I was crying out of fear I was going to lose my leg, and my mother was crying, too. My father sat by my side and held my hand, because whenever I was hurting, he was hurting too. My father tried to convince me that I was going to hold onto my leg *and* my life. He said the doctors knew what they were doing and would never let anything bad happen to me. But if I refused to let the doctor amputate, we all had to face the reality that I might die. It was a distinct possibility. When a doctor says he may have to take your leg to save your life, he's telling you, Hey, you're *close*, son.

"My parents tried to console me by saying it was not going to happen," Jeff said. "But they said that if the doctor did have to amputate, we would get through it and life would go on. My parents were always optimistic. But I was bullheaded about it. I said, 'Well, if he has to take my leg, then he might as well let me die.' I was more scared of losing my leg than of losing my life."

Jeff had always played sports with two legs. What satisfied him more than anything else in life was absolute freedom of movement. As far as he was concerned, Dr. Lockhardt had no shot at taking his leg, however much it rotted away. The leg belonged to him, it was his exclusive property, and it was going to stay put, attached to the rest of him, because under no circumstances was he about to surrender his identity as an athlete. Take his leg? They had to be kidding. He knelt on that leg behind the plate. He planted that leg before swinging the bat. He stepped forward with that leg before throwing the ball. He needed that leg! Dr. Lockhardt and his surgical team had better get to the bottom of the problem—and pronto—because nobody was taking his left leg.

Jeff was wheeled into surgery, with Bob and Verda Banister waiting in a corridor outside. The parents paced and looked down at the tiled floor, saying nothing to each other. Again Dr. Lockhardt probed the ankle and again he found the worrisome speck, about the size of a pencil head, that previous procedures had failed to extricate. He still strongly suspected that the speck had caused all the trouble. Now, for the first time, he reached toward the spot with his tweezers and firmly took it out. With the speck gone, Dr. Lockhardt decided that amputating the leg would be unnecessary after all. Then he sutured the gaping wound in the ankle.

Jeff endured six operations on his leg, receiving treatment in the hospital for four months straight. "I must have stayed in there three months before someone could come visit me without a mask on," he said. New tissue finally grew back around his ankle, and the doctors grafted skin onto the hole in his leg and prepared to send him home. As he recuperated from the trauma, Jeff picked up his daydreaming where he had left off. "I kept thinking about what I was going to do after I got out of the hospital," he said. "I told myself that as soon as I got out, I was going to be an athlete again. I told myself that as long as I had both my legs, I was going to play baseball again."

The day before Jeff left the hospital, he consulted with Dr. Lockhardt. His first question was, "Hey, how long before I can get out of here and play?"

"Play?" the doctor asked. As the hospital specialists had already informed Jeff, calcium deposits had clogged his ankle and limited his range of motion. It appeared that he would have difficulty walking, much less pivoting and sliding and kneeling and everything else he would have to do to hit and play catcher and run the bases.

"Yeah," Jeff pressed, "when am I going to be able to get back out on the baseball field?"

"You're crazy. You're not going to be able to run."

"I'll run, all right. First I'll walk, and then I'll run, and then I'll play baseball."

Dr. Lockhardt paused at this presumption and stiffened in his chair, ready to take umbrage at this forecast. The doctor had a crusty, stern manner, but with an overlay of compassion—quite similar, Jeff thought, to his own father. "Okay," the doctor said. "Whenever you think you're able to get back out there, you should get back out there."

And on that note, Jeff left the hospital.

❦ ❦ ❦

Out of the institution, away from the drugs and backless gowns and bedpans, Jeff still had to cope with his immobility, and he grew depressed. Back at home, Bob and Verda refused to let Jeff dwell on whatever apprehensions he might let fester about his life. If his parents had a message, it was that Jeff was going to have to come to terms with the challenges of rehabilitation.

"You can only go in one of two directions," Jeff's father told him. "You can either give up or you can go on."

Jeff recalled, "I always knew that it was not going to end like this, that life had much more in store for me. Nothing in the world was going to make my baseball career end like this."

He hobbled around the Banister home on crutches and performed the exercises the doctors gave him to do. He bent his ankle forward and back and turned it around in circles, trying to regain some degree of flexibility, and it hurt. Acting as his own doctor and nurse he daily withdrew the bandages packed into his ankle to allow drainage, then redressed it. The hole, once the size of a baseball, shrank in half, then within weeks, to the diameter of a nickel.

Jeff took school lessons from a private tutor at home every morning, then went out for a walk around the block. Because his legs had atrophied somewhat, he stepped slowly and gingerly. Eventually, as he felt stronger and more confident, he tried some light jogging. He would jog a few hundred yards, then walk, then jog some more. By the summer, his rehabilitation had progressed enough for him to start running flat-out. His father took him to the high school football field to run some wind sprints.

Jeff had a close friend, Greg Roach, who played football. Growing up together, they had formed a pact stipulating that they would both become professional athletes—Greg in football, Jeff in baseball—and live next door to each other. Now they renewed this pledge and began training together. They would run four or five miles together, loosening up and breaking a sweat, and then stop off at the one gym in town. The facility was basically a shack with a weight room. You never saw the owner, but you had a key and out front was a mailbox that you slipped your dues into each month. The gym was so hot and cramped and generally low-rent that local athletes dubbed it "The Sweatbox." There Jeff would hit the weight machines and work the legs, doing leg curls, leg presses, and leg extensions, all to strengthen the muscles, ligaments, and tendons in his left leg. "I would just pound it to death because my loss of nerve tissue in the ankle gave me an advantage: no pain," Jeff said. During these sessions, Jeff and Greg would talk about someday being pro. And if Jeff slacked off, Greg got on his case.

The ankle stiffened and swelled after every workout, and Jeff would have to ice it down. But otherwise, everything seemed to be working out fine. Dr. Lockhardt checked him out every two weeks. The boy returned to living a normal life. Then, early in the summer (he had skipped baseball that spring), he had an apparent relapse.

Jeff and Greg were driving trucks for a moving company, hauling furniture to and from warehouses. One afternoon, Jeff felt weak and feverish and went home early. As he took off his pants, he saw long red streaks running down his left leg from his thigh to his foot. He showed his parents the abnormality and they drove him to the hospital. Oh no, everyone thought, not again.

Dr. Lockhardt found that the lymph glands in the left leg, appearing striped as if marked with red crayon, had grown inflamed and infected. He suspected osteomyelitis, an infectious inflammation of the bone marrow, in Jeff's lower left leg. This new complication had given rise to not one cyst but several, all growing in the ankle. Dr. Lockhardt performed his seventh operation on the leg to extract the cysts. Jeff, taking antibiotics, stayed in the hospital for 18 days. He was then stitched up and sent home. Finally and unequivocally, Jeff was in the clear. It was the last time he saw a doctor for the treatment of cancer.

❦ ❦ ❦

In January of his senior year, Jeff tried out for the high school baseball team. He had gone without playing the game since his freshman year, about two-and-a-half years. He still had a bazooka arm, but when it came to swinging the bat and fielding, Jeff had gotten rusty. In the tryouts, he felt more awkward than the long layoff had led him to expect he might. Batting, he often swung and missed, and, if he made contact, the ball hardly rocketed toward the fences, as before. Fielding, he felt ham-handed and muffed plays that previously had come easily to him. Running, he suffered a slight limp due to his still-unstable ankle. All he had to fall back on was his arm, still an instrument vaguely reminiscent of a catapult with radar. But Jeff gave it his all for Coach Bruce Marshall. If his ankle prevented him from shifting his body to block an errant pitched ball, Jeff would snare the toss with his bare hand.

Marshall visited Jeff at his house the night before he was to make the final cut for the baseball team that season. Coach and player, seated in the front yard, settled in for a long talk. Marshall told a story about a guy who had tried out for the team without having played for two years. The guy looked out of practice and was in danger of missing the cut. The coach said he sure hated to cut him from the team because it was his senior year and, besides, his mom and dad were teachers at the school, but he had to make room in his program for some younger kids. It immediately became obvious to Jeff that Marshall was talking about him. More to the point, the coach was warning Jeff of the painful decision he was about to carry out, explaining the circumstances and, by serving notice, trying to let him down easy.

"I know who you're talking about, Coach," Jeff said. "Just give me one more day to try out. That's all I want. One more day to show you what I can do."

Marshall nodded sure, what the heck. But Jeff could tell the coach was humoring him.

The next day, Jeff went out to the high school baseball field and proved the coach wrong, surprising even himself. "Suddenly," he said, "I could hit. I could catch." He bombed the ball into the nether reaches of the outfield and vacuumed every pitch thrown to him behind the plate. "It was like something had happened overnight," he said. "A 180-degree turnaround. I looked like a totally different ballplayer than I had."

Marshall came over to Jeff after the tryout and said, "Where did all this come from?"

The youngster had no idea.

Jeff made the team on the strength of his dramatically improved performance on the last day of tryouts. His teammates, knowing his medical history full well, called him Robocatcher. That spring, he hit respectably for the school, posting a .250 batting average. But defensively, he proved to be an invaluable asset. Of course, he was grateful just to be playing. He believed he was a better player than his statistics suggested. But now, with the season almost over, he also found himself bedeviled by doubts about himself. It occurred to him that maybe he was never going to be as good as before. Maybe the seven operations on his cancerous leg and the long layoff had set him back too far in his quest to go on to the major leagues.

What bothered him more than any other problem was that, although he still viewed himself as a slugger, he had gone through the whole season without a home run. This conspicuous omission from the record book seemed to signal the onset of his demise. But then something special happened. In the last game of the season, his team was pitted against its cross-town rivals, Texas City, in an away game at the biggest stadium in the league. From home plate it was 360 feet down the lines and 420 feet to straightaway center, above standard distances for most major-league stadiums. Jeff came up for what would most assuredly be his last at-bat of the season.

He cracked a drive to left-center field, and it was a serious piece of ballistics. In LaMarque, he knew as soon as the ball jumped off the bat, the shot would have cleared the fence by about 90 feet. Now he ran to first base and watched the flight of the ball and wondered whether it was going out. The ball landed on top of the left-center fence, about 380 feet away. He lost sight of it. It seemed to have bounced over for a home run. Jeff looked at the first-base umpire and, sure enough, the ump signaled a home run.

Jeff leaped straight up, bum ankle and all, and sprinted around the bases as if roasting from a hot foot. He hopped with glee as he rounded second and third, and, after he stomped on home plate, he caught some stiff, slamming high fives from his teammates. Jeff figured that if you're going to cap off a season—hell, if you're going to wrap a ribbon around a comeback from cancer—you might as well do it with a home run.

"If that ball had bounced back onto the field of play," he recalled, "I might have just said to myself, okay, I was just a good high-school player, nothing more, nothing special. I ought to forget about the majors. But that's not what happened. No, sir. The ball *did* go over. It hit the fence and bounced over. And when that ball turned out to be a home run, something happened inside of me. I *knew*. I knew I was a baseball player. And meant to be a *professional* baseball player. It convinced me that I was going to keep trying, going to give baseball everything I had."

That home-run blast gilded his final high-school season. "I was exactly where I wanted to be for the first time in such a long time, and the next morning I could actually look at myself in the mirror," he said. "That was definitely the turning point in my career. It gave me an even stronger desire to be a professional, and I decided that I was going to do whatever I could, by whatever means possible, to fulfill that dream."

But the comeback would turn out to be short-lived, his sense of success premature. Jeff had no idea that he was about to come closer than ever to dying.

❦ ❦ ❦

In October 1985 Jeff was going to sit out a baseball game between his team, Lee Junior College of Baytown, Texas, and Dallas Northwood Junior College. But a scout for the New York Yankees called the coach at Lee the night before the game. He had watched the Banister kid all fall and wanted to see him before the winter draft for junior college players. The scout asked whether the coach planned to play him. To oblige, the coach put Jeff behind the plate for a few innings.

Jeff acquitted himself well in front of the Yankee scout, rapping out two singles and throwing out a couple of runners from behind the plate. His parents happened to be in the stands, along with his sister and a close friend.

In the sixth inning, with runners on second and third and one out, Lee led by several runs. Jeff hunched behind the plate as a batter lofted a twisting fly ball into shallow right field. Not deep enough for the runner on third base to break for home, Jeff thought. But the runner on third must have felt lucky because he bolted for the plate and came charging down the line. The right fielder caught the pop-up flat-footed and flung the ball toward home. The throw swerved off-line, about 10 feet from home plate. Jeff homed in to catch the throw along the third-base line, swivel around to his left and tag the runner out in one fluid motion.

The peg came skidding in and Jeff knelt down to play the short-stop, parked smack in the middle of the base path as the runner buffaloed toward him. He figured the runner would try to slow down or swerve around him. Big mistake. The runner never hit the brakes or changed course. Instead, he crashed flush into Jeff and popped him good. His knee smashed into the top of Jeff's head and split his skull wide open. Blood poured down his face mask. The collision sent Jeff sprawling to the field on his side. The runner crossed the plate for the score and came out of the accident with only a bruised knee.

The survivor of seven surgeries for bone cancer lay on the baseball field, motionless and unconscious, in front of his mother, his father, his sister, his friend, and the scout from the New York Yankees who had come to the game specially to see him in action.

"I knew I was hurt really bad," Jeff recalled. "It was like I had hit my funny bone. First my whole body felt like nothing, and then it was tingling. Really tingling. Everything seemed to go into slow motion, even the sound. I felt like I was in a tunnel, in a time warp. It was like my whole life was passing before me. I saw everything I'd ever gone through, all the baseball games. It seemed that from the time I got hit it took forever for someone to get to me. A whole lifetime."

The Lee baseball coach came over to Jeff and cupped his hand over his forehead to try to stop the blood from dripping into his eyes. Jeff had the uncanny sensation that even though his back was facing the stands, he could see his mother and father and sister and everyone else screaming for him to get off the ground. "I thought I was dead," he said.

Jeff tried to move, tried to stand. "I can't feel anything," he told the coach. "I can't get up."

"Just stay put," the coach said. The umps came over and the coach called Bob Banister out on the field. The father knelt beside his son.

"Did I get him out?" Jeff asked, referring to the runner.

His father shrugged, unwilling to answer no. Then Jeff took a stab at levity. He had started chewing tobacco after high school, and his father had urged him to quit. But Jeff insisted that the habit went hand in hand with baseball and kept working that chaw in his jaw. Now, lying there with his limbs still and blood spurting from his head, Jeff seized the opportunity to needle his father. "I suppose," Jeff croaked, "that none of this would have happened if I'd listened to you and stopped chewing tobacco."

The father chuckled gruffly.

Then the son, his tone suddenly grave, repeated, "I can't feel anything." Again he tried to get up, and again he slumped back down to the ground. As Jeff recalled, he knew then that something was "bad wrong."

The catcher remained immobile for 30 minutes as paramedics tried to identify the problem and bring him around. "I could feel nothing," Jeff said. "I tried to move my arms and my legs. Nothing."

Then an ambulance fishtailed onto the field, spreading clouds of dust. The paramedics scooped Jeff up onto a stretcher, strapped him down, and sped off to a hospital in nearby Alvin, Texas. A doctor in the emergency room wove 13 stitches through the gash in his head and took X-rays. "It's a bruised spinal column," he declared to Jeff. "Everything's going to be okay."

Then the doctor bustled over to tell Bob and Verda Banister and the paramedics that the boy had better get to a neurosurgeon. Fast. The comment about a bruised spinal column was all sugar-coating, earmarked for Jeff. The doctor, concerned that his young patient might panic, was reluctant to tell what had really happened.

The ambulance bearing the 21-year-old burned rubber out of Alvin and headed north, toward Galveston County Memorial Hospital. The emergency room doctor called ahead to alert the neurosurgeon to meet the Banisters immediately on arrival.

The neurosurgeon didn't tell Jeff what had happened either, but he told his parents. He steered the Banisters to a quiet corridor, unaware that here were a mother and father whose son had almost lost his leg to cancer two years earlier. He imparted the news with all the delicacy he could muster. All the parents could remember was the phrase "damage to the spinal cord." An X-ray and CAT scan revealed the specifics: three crushed vertebrae, the fifth, sixth, and seventh cervical vertebrae in his neck.

Jeff had broken his neck. He was paralyzed.

"Deep down inside I knew," Jeff said.

The day Jeff checked in at Galveston Memorial, the neurosurgeon told his parents and the other physicians and nurses involved in his care that, given his delicate condition, the young man would probably not last the night. If—as he lay there in traction, his head clamped into place by screws on either side—Jeff so much as coughed or sneezed, or if an orderly accidentally bumped into his bed, that was all it would take to push him over the precipice. It would all be over.

"Nobody told me about this," Jeff recollected. "Nobody said a word. It was all a big secret. Nobody told me anything until much later."

Even so, Jeff sensed something was wrong—bad wrong, as he would put it—because nobody would touch him, not even his mother. Nobody, neither nurses nor orderlies, would even come close to his bed. The bed was specially rigged inside a contraption that looked like a Ferris wheel. Two giant circles surrounded the bed, crosswise and lengthwise, enabling the patient to be rotated without his body actually moving. Tilting the bed forward or back would lift him upright or flatten him out; a nudge to the left or right would turn him on his side. All well and good, except that this amusement park ride—high-tech advancement though it is—induced in Jeff a level of motion sickness. Tilting the bed made him dizzy and nauseated.

The next morning, Jeff awoke in this circular electric bed, still alive, evidently against all odds. The neurosurgeon told Bob and Verda that his survival through the night was a miracle. The hospital had seen patients with significantly less severe spinal column damage who had died within 24 hours.

❧ ❧ ❧

Now came time for Jeff to once again enter a brightly lighted place he knew all too well and had prayed never to see again, the operating room. A nurse shaved his head, gently unharnessed him from traction, and carted him down a hall for surgery. Dr. Leroy Lockhardt, who had handled all seven leg operations, now stepped to the fore again. He cut into Jeff's back and extracted fragments of shattered vertebrae from his neck and shaped the bones into makeshift vertebrae, then inserted prostheses to shore up his spine. Dr. Lockhardt painstakingly plucked bone chips—the shrapnel from the crash—out of his spinal column. The procedure lasted four hours.

The first week back in the hospital Jeff thought he had had it, and a gloom as oppressive as any he had ever felt descended on him. He lay rigidly in traction, his head braced in one position, and refused to let the nurses open the curtains to his room. If the curtains were pulled open, he would see the world outside the hospital. He would see the sun and want to leave and play baseball. And wanting to go outside would remind him that he was stuck inside, in the chilled, clinical atmosphere of a hospital, and that he remained unable to move, let alone walk. He would rather rest, free of such painful distraction, in the twilight cool of his hospital room, burrowed inside his thoughts.

Dr. Lockhardt warned Jeff that he might be paralyzed permanently, and in that event would need a wheelchair. Jeff figured it was really only a matter of time before it was all over. Sometimes his eyes would snap open at night, and the room would be dark, and he would have no feeling in his body. He would wonder whether he was awake or dreaming or perhaps had already died.

"I dreamt I was sinking into this huge hole, and I tried to get out," Jeff recalled. "But I never could, and when I woke, it would feel as if I'd died, and I would be petrified." Later, toward dawn, Jeff would fall back into a restless sleep and dream again. In his dreams he would replay the accident that had brought him back to the hospital. Every night he dreamed about the collision along the third-base line. In the dream he would try to see himself sidestep the runner sprinting for home, try to avoid breaking his neck. But it never worked. He always got nailed. He had thought he was inside the third-base line, on the grass. But instead he had parked himself on the dirt, directly on the base path. And that made him fair game for a runner looking to score. No dream could change what had happened.

In his waking moments, Jeff never begrudged the runner his run scored. "It was just good, hard, clean baseball," he said. "He could have gone around me. But he did what he had to do."

However long Jeff might lie in traction, though, nothing could handcuff his imagination. He would fantasize about baseball, just as he had during his cancer, almost as if it were an exercise prescribed for him. He would visualize all the ballfields on which he had played over the years, from the sandlots and the corner parks to the well-groomed diamonds at LaMarque High School and Bobby Beach Stadium. "I still had baseball on the brain," he said. "I would think about being on the baseball field, and it always looked the same. The sun was always shining. The grass was always bright green. The stands were always filled with smiling fans. In my mind baseball always looked pretty. And as long as I was in the hospital, I saw baseball as my escape."

The first surgery went well. Jeff regained sensation in both arms and his left leg. But he still had no feeling in his right leg. And he still lay on his back, still in the grip of traction, his head still held stationary by screws.

Through it all, he reflected on his fight with cancer. It was inevitable now, back in the hospital, that he do so.

"I'd been there before," Jeff said, "and that almost made it easier for me. I pretty much knew what I was up against. I knew I had my back up against the wall. But somebody had rung the bell and it was time for me to come out fighting again. In that situation I could go in one of two directions. I could either go down or I could start climbing. And knowing I had been there before, that I had climbed out from the cancer, gave me confidence that I could get through it again. That confidence became the backbone of my recovery."

Susan Jones, a nurse, lent a hand, too. She saw a Jeff Banister no one else saw. He might strike a pose in front of his parents and teammates and friends—the disabled athlete down but never out, jaw jutting out heroically in the face of challenge—but Jones knew better. She knew that his heart was as broken as his neck. She saw him panic over his paralysis and she saw him cry. "She would come in when I was screaming and hollering in my hospital room all by myself and comfort me," Jeff said. "She did what my parents did when they were there. Talked to me, helped me just by being there. Once she even cried along with me."

After a week, Dr. Lockhardt operated on Jeff again. This surgery resembled the previous one, except that the doctor ventured in through the front, not the back. He withdrew bone from the front and back of Jeff's hip, a graft, and strung the bone around the three vertebrae that the collision had pulverized. In so doing, he wired the vertebrae from both above and below, fusing the spine together. An elaborate work of architecture.

Afterward, Jeff regained feeling in his right leg. He was no longer paralyzed. He had lain in traction for 10 days. Ten days in the Ferris wheel bed, imprisoned in inertia. Ten days with the curtains closed, dark dreams taunting his thoughts late every night. Dr. Lockhardt had now saved his life twice.

No sooner had Jeff come out of traction than the staff replaced his hospital gown with a new outfit: a hard-plastic body cast. The enclosure extended from the top of his head to the small of his back, molded around his belly, chin, and neck, all tightly secured with Velcro straps. Now all Jeff had to do was learn to walk again.

❦ ❦ ❦

One morning, two occupational therapists, both specialists in rehabilitation, came to introduce themselves to Jeff in his room. One pressed a button to tilt the bed upright, making Jeff dizzy and queasy, while the other placed an aluminum walker alongside the bed. Together, they strapped a belt around his middle and hoisted him to a sitting position with his feet dangling off the side of the bed and the walker right in front of him.

"What are you all doing?" Jeff said. "What's this? I don't need this walker." He thought, They've got to be crazy. This is insane.

"Go ahead," a therapist said. "Use the walker. It's okay."

"I don't need it. I don't need a walker."

"Trust us," the therapist said. "You're going to need this walker and you're going to need us."

Upright for the first time in more than a week, Jeff still felt squeamish. But he had to try to walk, because only after he took some steps could he accelerate to a run and hope to make the grade in sprinting from home to first. He waited at the side of the bed until he felt he could get on his feet. He waited a long time because he dreaded a failure now, after almost losing his leg and then coming within a whisker of dying from a broken neck.

Jeff clutched the walker with sweaty palms and boosted himself off the bed, trying to stand. Each therapist supported him by the elbow. I can do it, Jeff thought. Walking is easy. I've walked since I was a baby.

Then he collapsed back onto the bed.

His body had forgotten all its lessons. He would have to start with the simple act of standing and graduate to walking. He would need a course in remedial movement. "That was a major shock," Jeff said. "I had to try to perform the simplest tasks, the tasks you take for granted, like sitting up on the side of a bed and getting up and walking across the room. I had never had to have somebody help me out of bed. But here I was, needing to hold on to a walker and have someone help me do it. I have never tried anything in my life harder than taking those first steps. I was upset about having somebody help me walk. I cried like a baby."

Finally, he stood from the bed and, trembling, held the walker. His brain told his feet to move, but his feet declined to pay attention. He gripped the walker to steady himself and took a step, the therapists guiding him from both sides, and then he took another step. He took about five steps and then, exhausted, he had to slide back into bed. "It made me feel better to move again, but I also realized how far I had to go," Jeff said. "I had to go back to square one."

By chance, Dr. Lockhardt happened to come in at that telling moment. With a keen sense of strategy designed to motivate his patient, the doctor told Jeff the news he had so carefully concealed from him at the beginning: that nobody had expected him to make it through the first night at Galveston Memorial. The news brought everything into perspective for Jeff. He had complained about the difficulty of walking, the indignity of relying on therapists to transport himself five steps, without knowing how close he had come to reaching the end of the line. And now he realized he had no right to complain.

"When Dr. Lockhardt told me the true story, it kind of sobered me up," Jeff said. "I realized that at least I was still alive. I might not have been able to walk, not yet anyway, but at least I was there, living and breathing."

At this news, Jeff turned to nurse Susan Jones. "I think it's about time I saw the sun again," he said. She understood: He wanted her to pull open the curtains to his room. She did so, and golden shafts of sunlight came showering in. Get me the hell out of here, he thought. I'm ready to go. Ready to live again.

Jeff remained in Galveston County Memorial Hospital for four-and-a-half months. The stack of medical bills for his broken neck was five inches thick, the expenses so astronomical that Lee Junior College had to find a new insurance company. The first surgery on his neck left him with a four-inch scar, about a quarter-inch wide, across his collarbone from shoulder to shoulder. The second, more extensive operation stamped him with a more memorable lifetime imprint: a six-inch, zipperlike scar, two inches wide—like the track from a bicycle tire—from the base of his skull to the middle of his shoulder blades. He would leave the hospital tattooed with scars.

But before Dr. Lockhardt let him go, Jeff asked the doctor the same question he had posed nearly two years earlier, on his release from cancer treatment. "Can I get back to playing baseball now?" he wanted to know.

This time the answer from Lockhardt came back as harsh as the teeth on a buzz saw. "You're crazy," he said matter-of-factly.

But then he had second thoughts. Lockhardt had seen the kid come back before, from no fewer than seven operations, and for bone cancer at that. Could anyone write off Robocatcher?

"Then again, who am I to tell you no?" Dr. Lockhardt said. "Who am I to say, no, you'd better not even try to get out there and play? You're just going to do it anyway, so what difference does it make what I say to you? But I just want you to realize something. If you get hit again like you got hit before, either you're going to get up and walk away or they're going to bury you. You'd better be prepared to live with that knowledge."

Jeff thanked the doctor for his candor. Dr. Lockhardt was right: Jeff had already made up his mind what to do. Only the details remained.

Bob and Verda brought him home from the hospital. Jeff, still encased in his body cast, shuffled along, herky-jerky, with his walker. His parents piloted him through the front door and into his bedroom to rest for a spell. They, too, were worn out, and tucked themselves into bed for a long, well-deserved nap.

As his parents slept, Jeff rolled around in bed. He was so happy to be home he could hardly lie still. He slithered to the side of his bed, boosted himself upright, and groped for his walker. He wanted to go outside. Outside was where the sun always shone and the grass always glinted bright green and the stands were always filled with smiling fans. Outside was where baseball happened. Jeff shambled out of his room and went out the front door into the noontime daylight.

Once in the front yard, he pulled over a light plastic lawn chair from the porch and set it down on the grass. No longer was he in the hospital, with doctors and nurses shuttling in and out with trays of medication and fresh sheets. He was home again. Jeff leaned his head back in the lawn chair with the sun beaming down on his face, pale from so many months inside, and felt the warmth seep into his skin and soothe him.

He decided to go for a walk. Giddy with a sense of liberty, he reached for his walker and started out for a shuffle around the block.

Meanwhile, his mother woke up from her nap and went to check on Jeff in his bedroom. When she discovered him missing, Verda had no idea where her injured boy might have gone. She shook her husband awake. Together, the Banisters scoured the house for Jeff. No luck. Where could he have gone? Why would he leave like that, without even telling us? What if he falls?

Bolting from the front door, they saw the lawn chair, obviously moved from its previous location, and Verda started to panic. "Jeff!" she screamed. "*Jeff*! Where are you, Jeff! *Jeeeeff*!" The Banisters jumped into the family car, floored it out of the driveway, and took off around the block. A few hundred yards from the house, they spotted Jeff. He was hobbling gamely along with his walker, basking in his newly found freedom. They abruptly braked the car and asked Jeff to kindly explain his sudden, unannounced departure from the premises.

"I just wanted to go out for a walk," Jeff said. "I let you sleep because you were both so tired."

Perfect, his parents thought. We brought him home from the hospital sheathed in a body cast, able to ambulate thanks only to an aluminum walker, fresh from yet another brush with death, and he decides, while we're napping, that he just wants to go out for a walk. No warning. No note posted on the refrigerator door. No nothing. But as ticked off at this gumption as his parents were, they realized Jeff had meant no harm. They drove home and let him continue his walk. Jeff shuffled around the whole block before he came back.

"I must have scared the living fire out of my folks," Jeff said. "They were scared to death something had happened to me." Indeed. Something *had* happened. Jeff had gone for a walk. And in the process, he had taken his first steps toward yet another comeback.

After a year of rehab, during which his parents took turns feeding, changing, and bathing him, Jeff finally regained full movement in his back and neck. He grew to 6 feet, 2 inches tall and built himself to a hard, sinewy 210 pounds, almost as big as his dad. He wore a size 13 shoe, and his massive, meaty hands could easily palm a basketball. He moved like an athlete, shoulders straight back, with an air of pride and self-assurance sometimes mistaken for arrogance. He had the look of an all-American baseball player, a Boy Scout with advanced hormones. His blond hair was cropped short, his eyes sky-blue, and he had high cheekbones with a square jaw. In an old movie, he would have played the fighter pilot who wins the Purple Heart, marries a WAC, and always gives his mother flowers on her birthday.

Jeff returned to Lee Junior College, before accepting a baseball scholarship to the University of Houston, and graduated from there with a degree in sports administration. Everyone pleaded with him to quit catching and switch to a position where a collision was less likely. His parents and Dr. Lockhardt finally prevailed on him to try first base and then outfield for the Houston Cougars. But Jeff was miserable unless hunkered down behind the plate and took up catching afresh.

In the major-league baseball draft of June 1986, the Pittsburgh Pirates picked him in the 25th round, despite his being what most scouts termed an extreme medical risk. Jeff started with the Watertown Pirates, a minor league, single A team in upstate New York, and batted a meager .189 in a brief season. The next year he transferred to the Macon Pirates in Georgia, also a single A ball club, where he hit .270 with seven home runs and 70 runs batted in.

More than once, he found himself racing toward home plate and crashing into catchers. But it was no vendetta, no attempt at payback. That's how the game goes, he would think. Everyone knows it and accepts it. If you get hurt in the process, it's tough luck, pal.

Even so, the bone cancer had left its legacy. He still ran with a slight limp, still had to crouch behind the plate with his left heel raised an inch, awkwardly so, rather than flattened out. Dr. Lockhardt worried that the ankle might otherwise fuse permanently into the wrong angle and stop Jeff from bending or running for good. The outside of the ankle remained traumatized from seven operations to gouge out cysts. "I have no feeling there," Jeff said. "I feel no pain at all in my left ankle, sometimes just a vague pressure. I may spike the cleats on my right foot against my left ankle, or get hit on that ankle with a baseball, and I'll never know what happened until I see blood flying off the ankle and a big red blood spot on my sock."

Jeff rose through the minor-league circuit and joined the Harrisburg Senators, a double A team in Pennsylvania, for two seasons. He posted a .265 batting average with six homers and 40 RBI in his first year there and improved the next, batting .270 with 13 homers and 60 RBI. Jeff showed such consistency that the Pirates organization promoted him to the Buffalo Bisons, its Class AAA farm club in upstate New York. There, in the summer of 1991, facing even stiffer competition, he was hitting .276 with 14 home runs and 65 RBI.

For Jeff Banister, the best seemed yet to come.

❦ ❦ ❦

On Tuesday, July 22, 1991, Jeff reclined on a sofa checking out ESPN on the tube with his Buffalo Bisons roommate Jeff Richardson when the phone trilled. Jeff had expected a call from his wife, Karen, whom he had married in 1988. Richardson answered the phone, listened for two seconds, and turned to Banister.

"It's Terry," he said, referring to Buffalo manager Terry Collins. "It's the big leagues calling you up."

Oh, sure, Banister thought. Richardson had a habit of playing pranks on him, especially jokes about getting The Call from the majors. Richardson would answer the phone and, with a straight face, say to Banister, "Oh, it's for you. It's Jim Leyland [manager of the Pittsburgh Pirates], and he wants to bring you up right away." But it was always someone else calling, maybe his mother or his wife or a friend, never The Call. Richardson just went in for good-natured teasing and Banister, now wise to the routine, stopped falling for the fake-out.

But Richardson insisted. "Jeff," he said again, "it's Terry and it's really the big leagues calling you up."

"Yeah, right," Banister said. He took the phone and said hello, expecting to hear Karen answer. But it sounded just like Terry Collins.

"Jeff," the voice at the other end said, "I know how long you've waited for this phone call."

"Who the hell is this?" Banister asked.

"Well, Jeff," the voice explained, "Don Slaught [starting catcher for the Pirates] got hurt tonight, and he's on the 15-day disabled list with a pulled rib-cage muscle, and the Pirates want you to fly out to Pittsburgh tomorrow. You're going to the majors, man."

"Come on, who the hell is this?" Jeff demanded. "This is not a good joke to play on somebody."

"No, Jeff, this is no joke. This really is Terry Collins. Don Slaught really got hurt, and you're really going to the big leagues. They need you to report tomorrow."

"All right now, I'm getting ready to hang up the phone. Who the hell is this?" Banister kept thinking, It sure sounds like Terry Collins.

"Jeff, listen. This really is Terry. I'm proud and happy to give you this message. It could hardly have happened to a better person. You have to be at the airport tomorrow morning for a 10:20 flight to Pittsburgh. They'll have a plane ticket all ready for you at the front desk. I'm not sure how long you'll be with the Pirates because we're not sure how bad Slaught is hurt. But we are sure that they want you there. The Pirates have a doubleheader coming up, and you'd better be ready to play."

Banister, at 26, a four-and-a-half-year veteran of the minors, was older than most minor-league players. He knew that the more years you stayed in the minors, the further away seemed your chances of making the Majors.

He was still not buying the phone call. Maybe Richardson had put another teammate up to the shenanigan.

But Banister had a plan. The next day, Buffalo was scheduled to take a flight to Oklahoma City for a game. So he had to go to the airport anyway. If the message from Terry Collins was legitimate, if he had really received The Call, he would find out at the Buffalo airport when he picked up his ticket. A plane was going to take him either to Oklahoma City or to Pittsburgh. He just wanted to see that airplane ticket. From there he would play it by ear.

Jeff slept that night as if reclining on thorns. If the Pirates really were in the cards for him, he was loath to risk sleeping through the alarm the next morning and missing his flight. He rolled around in bed reviewing his baseball life from Little League to the Class AAA Buffalo Bisons. He pondered the cysts that kept growing back and the crash that had smashed his vertebrae. He had spent a total of one year of his life in the hospital, occupying so many of those hours daydreaming about making the bigs. It had all come down to the destination printed on an airline ticket.

The next morning, Jeff rode to the airport with his fellow Bisons. He kept his mouth shut rather than risk being branded a laughingstock over this likely gag. He approached the ticket counter at the airport. "Jeff Banister," he said, identifying himself. "I believe you have a ticket for me." He was handed an envelope, and opened it quickly.

The ticket said: PITTSBURGH.

Jeff thought, Hey, this is for real.

The ticket also said: FIRST-CLASS. Jeff had always flown coach. The first-class section was what he passed through to get to his seat. Now he parked himself in a seat wider than he was accustomed to, with the flight attendants smiling more broadly and attending more closely to his whims than had ever happened before. He decided that, as long as he was flying first-class, he might as well partake of its pleasures, and ordered an omelet and orange juice. What was special, though, was that his juice came not in a plastic cup but in a glass, and that his breakfast tray came with salt and pepper in regular shakers rather than those pop-open packets. Even before he got to Pittsburgh, he had tasted a hint of the major-league life.

I just want to get to Pittsburgh as quickly as I possibly can, he thought as he rode first-class. I just want to sign that contract and see my uniform hanging in the locker room before somebody changes his mind.

The flight lasted about an hour. But the trip defied conventional measurement in miles or minutes. The ride really took him four-and-a-half years. It carried him from the Buffalo Bisons to the Pittsburgh Pirates, the Pirates of Roberto Clemente and Willie Stargell and Dave Parker, the World Series champions of 1960 and 1971 and 1979, and now, in 1991, pennant contenders again.

❦ ❦ ❦

Everyone Jeff initially encountered in Pittsburgh called him either "Sir" or "Mr. Banister." In the Hilton downtown, where the Pirates had booked him a room, the manager behind the front desk instantly recognized his name, knew he was associated with the Pirates, and called him Sir. The bellman who hoisted his bags and escorted him upstairs to a lovely room addressed him with equal formality. He had never stayed in a Hilton before, least of all as a member of the Pittsburgh Pirates. Yes, Mr. Banister. Certainly, Mr. Banister. Of course, Mr. Banister. Red-carpet treatment for the kid from the oil depot of LaMarque.

This is like a dream, Jeff thought.

In the hotel room, he left his bags unpacked, eager to take care of business. Never know when somebody might change his mind, he thought. Maybe the Pirates will see they made a mistake. Maybe they meant to call up a different Jeff Banister.

He walked briskly over to Three Rivers Stadium and strode into the front office, where he met general manager Larry Doughty. "We're happy you're here," Doughty said. "You know Slaught's on the disabled list. We can't guarantee how long you'll be here. So just get ready."

"I'm ready, Mr. Doughty," Jeff said.

A secretary typed out his contract with the Pirates and set the pages down in front of Jeff. The terms called for the then-minimum major-league salary: $100,000 a year. Not bad as raises go. With Buffalo, he was pulling down $1,700 a month, one-fifth as much. "I'd never seen so many zeros next to my name," Jeff recalled. He signed the contract without pause. As far as he was concerned, he would have played for the Pirates for meal and motel money.

He went around the corner from the front office to the clubhouse. Approaching the lockers, he saw a Pittsburgh Pirates jersey hanging on the door, bearing number 28. Big black letters stitched on the back said: JEFF BANISTER. Around game time, wearing the Pirates uniform, Jeff headed through the hallway that led to the home-team dugout. Seated there in the dugout, he could look across the bench at his teammates Andy Van Slyke and Barry Bonds and Bobby Bonilla. From this vantage point he could see the field and the night sky and all the hometown fans waiting for the contest with the Atlanta Braves. And that's when it all sank in for Jeff.

I'm here. I'm finally here.

Pirates manager Jim Leyland started Mike LaValliere at catcher, and that was okay with Jeff. He had waited his whole life to make the pros, and now he could wait another few innings or even until the next game to get in there and take his cuts.

In the seventh inning, with one out and nobody on base, the Pirates led by seven runs and seemed to have the game well in hand. Pitcher Doug Drabek was scheduled to bat, but Leyland waved Jeff over and told him to go pinch-hit. Jeff felt his heart pounding away. The Pirates' announcer introduced Banister to the crowd, but the rookie was so caught up in rushing to find a bat for himself that he missed hearing his name echo out over the field. Now he strode toward home plate and dug in against Atlanta pitcher Dan Petrie. Jeff knew that his family—his wife Karen, his mother, his sister Carey, his grandmother Genevieve, his

Uncle Tony and Aunt Ellen, his nephews Sean and Joshua, and his niece Shelly—was home in LaMarque watching the game on TBS. Jeff thought, I just want to get three swings and look like I belong.

Petrie fired the first pitch high and hard, almost clipping Jeff on the chin. Welcome to the big leagues, kid. That's what the pitch seemed to say. Jeff stabbed his cleats into the dirt and took his stance again: upright, legs close together and slightly bent, bat held at the very end. The next pitch sailed in right down the pipe, and Jeff swung hard and missed. He tugged at his jersey, pulled his helmet down low and stepped in again. Petrie went into his windup. The pitch veered off low and away, and Jeff let it go. Two balls, one strike.

For the next pitch, Petrie delivered a fastball, clearly destined to be a strike. The ball sizzled in about knee-high and inside, a spot where Jeff happened to like a pitch. He lashed his bat around and struck the ball squarely, lining a shot into the gap between the shortstop and the third baseman. Jeff Treadway, the shortstop, scooted over to his right, backing up deep, out to the rim of the left field grass. The ball bounced once and kicked up hard. Treadway lunged for it backhanded, snaring it in the web of his glove, then planted himself and fired his peg to first.

Jeff ran down the first base line with every ounce of fuel in his soul, racing against the throw from short. He would have to do the job with his legs. How ironic that he would have to rely on his legs, especially the left leg, the leg almost cut off. The sprint seemed to take an eternity. But finally Jeff stomped on the bag and the ump hollered the call from down in his diaphragm.

Safe.

Jeff had beaten the throw by a step. He had himself a single, an infield single. He looked at the stands, where the fans cheered his hustle. The significance of the hit was altogether lost on the TBS announcer who called the game. Jeff stood on first base and looked around the field in a daze. The Pirates' first-base coach whistled for the umpire to get the ball for Jeff as a memento. I'm in the big leagues, Jeff thought. I'm on the Pirates, and we're playing Atlanta at Three Rivers Stadium, and it's on national television, and my family and friends are watching me, and I just got a base hit. "I've hit a lot of home runs, including some grand slams and some long balls, but that infield single was the best hit ever," Jeff said. "It was the best feeling I could ever imagine—like I was on the highest mountain. People have no idea how high a mountain I had to climb to get that single. Every dream I'd ever had had just come true. It made it all worth it."

That night CNN would air a highlight film from the game, won by the Pirates, 12–3. The announcer would say, "Jeff Banister made his major league debut Tuesday night and it was perfect. He came up as a pinch hitter and delivered a single. The significance here is that Jeff Banister just getting to play in a major league game was one of the more valiant accomplishments in baseball. Banister is a walking testimony to courage, having fought leg cancer, a broken neck, bad knees, and 12 operations, all in the last five years."

After the game, Jeff sat down on the bench in front of his locker in the clubhouse. Inside his locker he found the ball he had hit. Still in a stupor, he tried quietly to collect his thoughts. The moment he turned around, the privacy he preferred came abruptly to an end. The media mobbed him. Three TV cameras pointed at him, bright lights glared in his eyes, and a half-dozen microphones jabbed toward his mouth. Reporters bombarded him with questions left and right, scribbling his answers.

The questions gave him a headache, and the lights made his eyes smart. So much was going through his mind, and he wanted to reflect for just a moment more and try to figure it all out. He wanted his wife and his mother and the rest of his family there with him, if only to shield him from this onslaught of attention. With the media pressing against him, this jostling throng of strangers wanting free admission to his thoughts, Jeff suddenly felt alone and rattled.

But he hung in there. He stayed cool and answered the questions. He told the cameras and microphones and notebooks that he wanted to thank his family. What motivated him to fight catastrophic medical problems, he acknowledged, was a combination of his loving parents and the game of baseball. His family had stood behind him during his bleak days in the hospital, had visited him in the Ferris-wheel bed and had believed in his dream of a comeback.

The reporters asked manager Jim Leyland to comment on Banister. "If he never does anything else in baseball, the fact that he got here is incredible," Leyland said. "He is really an amazing young man. It's hard to think of anyone who has had to overcome more." A reporter asked the hard-boiled manager what it was about the win over Atlanta that brought him the most happiness. Leyland said, "Jeff Banister got to play—*and* he got a hit."

Back at the Hilton, the front desk had dozens of phone messages for Jeff, calls from his wife, his mother, all his friends from Texas. Everyone had seen his base hit. He went to his hotel room and again felt lonely, profoundly so. Never had he so much wanted to share a moment with those he loved. His family was back in LaMarque. His father had died in January 1988, and his grandfather Leon had passed away two weeks later, and Dr. Lockhardt was gone, too, all departing from his life within three months of one another. Jeff wanted to tell his Dad that he had gone to the majors and gotten a hit. "He would've congratulated me and told me he was the proudest father in the world," Jeff said. "But I know my dad was there with me that day. He still sees everything I do. He still walks with me."

His dream to play big-league baseball had survived bone cancer and a broken neck, had survived almost everything going wrong, bad wrong. But above all, Jeff felt grateful, grateful for being twice saved and twice blessed.

"If, after the game, I could have shouted to the world my thank you to my family, then it would have made everything just right," Jeff reflected. "My family believed in my dream, believed I would be a big leaguer. Especially my father. Nobody ever told me, 'You should forget about baseball. You should think about getting on with your life.' I've received second and third chances, and for that I thank God. I believe God instills in all of us certain values that enable us to survive. But my father and mother taught me a lesson, too—that being a good patient means always having hope. And with that base hit, I was finally able to say thank you."

Chapter 2

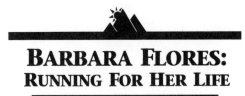

BARBARA FLORES:
RUNNING FOR HER LIFE

She went to the gynecologist expecting a routine physical exam. Take off the clothes, let the doctor look, get the good word. One, two, three. In and out. Same story as the last 23 annual checkups, starting back in 1966. But that's not quite what happened. Not this time. Not by a long shot.

In March 1989, Barbara Flores of Port Jefferson Station, New York, went in for a lunch-hour appointment feeling healthy and fit. The numbers looked good. Five-foot-seven, 125 pounds, at age 53. Long and lean, with her close-cropped light brown hair and deeply tanned face. Blood pressure, cholesterol, body fat: all low. An athlete, obviously. Nothing could go wrong—until, of course, something did.

Dr. Donald Bruhn, her gynecologist for 23 years, told her she had a blockage that prevented him from conducting a proper pelvic exam, and he would have to perform a sonogram and a magnetic resonance imaging test for a better view. Bruhn preferred to keep his suspicions to himself, but Barbara could tell something was going on. After 23 years, she could read him pretty well. She wanted to know: What was it, this blockage? Not sure, he said. But she forced the issue. Why leave your future hanging in the air, a balloon, untethered, near a needle? Might as well get right down to it. That's how Barbara had always lived, getting right down to it. Give me the bottom line, she said. Is it cancer?

It could be, Bruhn said. He wanted to tell her for sure. He wanted to be doctor-like and definitive, to give her either a thumbs up or a thumbs down, an unequivocal verdict. But he could only speculate. He had no bottom line for her yet. All he could say was maybe. Too bad, too. He liked Barbara, respected her intelligence, spirit and commitment to health.

"I thought this was dreadful," she recalled. "It was not anything I wanted to hear. I had no idea what it was all about, and I tried to clear my head. I had to calm myself down and finally, I said, 'Well, I better wait until the test results come out.'"

Bruhn asked her to come back two days later with her husband of 33 years, Ken, a flight engineer at Grumman Aerospace. This was it. It was like going to the principal. You knew you were going to get it now. She sat with Ken in the waiting room for 15 minutes, the longest quarter-hour either had ever endured. Then they walked into the private office holding hands, faces ashen and solemn, as if at a funeral. Bruhn laid it all on the line, getting right down to it.

"You have cancer. Ovarian cancer."

Yes, she heard him right. Cancer of the female reproductive glands. It was official now. The pelvic exam had revealed a large tumor on each ovary. If the growths spread to the bowels and other organs, she could die within a month. Bruhn needed to operate.

Barbara and Ken reacted with disbelief, had no idea what to say or ask. This was a family first, this malignancy. Hard to see the good there, hard to give ovarian cancer a positive spin. It was bad. Ovarian cancer was definitely bad. No getting around it. The news loomed over her like a wave, curled and crashed, and suddenly she was in over her head, her previous life gone, washed away.

Oh. Oh no. Oh, not this. Not now. Not me.

This was not supposed to happen. It was not what Barbara had in mind. She had planned to go home, run a few miles at the high school track, probably with Ken plodding along in her wake. They would eat dinner together, talk about the children, both grown up and out of the house now. Read the paper, catch the news on TV. Nod off early, before 10. Lights out, sweet dreams. The next day would dawn with promise, many tomorrows still ahead, the years beckoning to her. She would go on, nothing changed, everything perfect, just perfect. Her life was suffused with love, love of husband, son and daughter, friends, sports. But perfect never lasts.

Now everything would be different. She would need a new agenda. CAT scans. A laparotomy. A hysterectomy. Probably chemo. Then, almost certainly, she figured, death. No, not what she had in mind at all. And now Barbara began to miss her life, as though she had already died and said goodbye to everyone and everything: to Ken and the children, Kevin, 32, and Cindy, 29; to her best friend Pat; to the running, the swimming, the water skiing; and to the forays out onto the Long Island Sound in

"Summer Girl" a 25-foot Chris Craft—named after her, of course—to drop anchor and fish for blues and fluke. Soon it would all be gone, swept away in the riptide of cancer.

As they stared dumbfounded at Dr. Bruhn, Ken thought, Everything is being shot out from under us.

"I cried and Ken cried, and I told him I was going to die," Barbara recalled. "I said that right in front of my doctor. I said to Ken, 'I'm going to die and you'll be left all alone.' Then Ken and I cried some more. I told Dr. Bruhn I was afraid to go through with the surgery and the treatment because I had seen what had happened to my brother-in-law when he got cancer. I just rattled on and on, and Dr. Bruhn just sat and listened because he had known me a long time and he'd told this kind of news to patients before, and he said, 'Go ahead and say whatever you have to say.'"

They got in the car, the new spiffy white, two-seat CRX Honda—something else for her to miss, she realized. I might as well give it to Cindy, she thought. I won't need it because I won't be here. But before they reached home, she broke down crying again and Ken pulled into a parking lot. They sat there in the front seat with the motor off, hugging each other. Clutching just as they had in the 1950s at drive-ins and on dark, lonely roads. Only now Barbara sought not romance in his arms but sanctuary.

It hurt him to see her so sad. Hurt something terrible. It'll be okay, Ken whispered. You'll see. You'll be fine. Everything will work out. We'll get past this. We're going to be together a long time. He believed what he was saying, believed it because he wanted to believe it. He repeated the words and it became like a chant.

Back at home, they prayed. "I'm going to die," she sobbed. "No," Ken shushed her. "It'll be okay," he said in his steady voice. "Everything will be fine. We'll overcome this." In bed, they held each other tight, Ken whispering and shushing her in his last waking moments, and they drifted to sleep, still embracing. And as Barbara slept, she thought that maybe tomorrow she would go for a run.

❦ ❦ ❦

Ovarian cancer is among the deadliest of all cancers. Of every three women stricken with the disease, only one survives for five years or more. That means about 15,000 die every year from this condition, according to the American Cancer Society.

The disease is so often fatal for the simplest of reasons: all too frequently, the symptoms—and therefore the tumors—are detected too late. Patients pick up the warning signs, if at all, only after the disease is far along. Unfortunately, ovarian cancer seldom has any symptoms early on. Some women complain of persistent, otherwise unexplained stomach pain or discomfort, a sense of fullness, indigestion, or mild anorexia, but by then the disease is usually well-advanced. The disease can be difficult to detect in its earliest stages even in routine pelvic exams or through sophisticated diagnostic devices.

If an ovarian tumor is local, confined to the original site, the five-year survival rate is about 85 percent. If, however, the growth has spread to neighboring tissue and surrounding pelvic organs, the percentage plummets to about 40 percent. And if the malignancy has metastasized to far-off sites, such as those above the diaphragm, only about one in five patients live.

Cancer of the ovaries mainly affects women 40 to 70 years old, with most cases coming after menopause. The older the woman, the higher the risk. Women who have never given birth are two to three times more likely to develop the disease than those who have. The same goes for older women who've previously had breast, colorectal or endometrial cancer. Ovarian cancer can run in families: women who have two or more close relatives (mother, sister, daughter) with ovarian cancer have about a 50 percent chance of getting it themselves. Women with a history of either infertility, early menopause, a high-fat diet, exposure to asbestos or talc, a first pregnancy after age 30, or a chronic failure to ovulate also face higher-than-average risks.

Treatment of ovarian cancer depends on the extent of the tumor. An exploratory laparotomy is a procedure aimed at diagnosing and identifying its rate of growth. If the tumor is limited to the ovary, a hysterectomy, removal of the ovaries, is usually in order. When the cancer has spread, however, doctors may take out not only the ovaries, but also the fatty tissue near the pelvis, any other visible cancer tissue, and nearby lymph glands. After surgery, patients can receive either taxol, a drug derived from the bark of Pacific yew trees found mainly in the Northwest; chemotherapy (cyclophosphamide, cisplatin, hexamethylmelamine and doxorubicin); radiation; a bone marrow transplant; or a combination of the above.

The main test for finding ovarian cancer is the standard pelvic exam. By this method, the doctor inserts a speculum into the vagina to widen the opening and look at the canal and cervix; then by hand the doctor feels the uterus, ovaries, bladder, vagina, and rectum for any signs of abnormality or enlargement.

Unfortunately, by the time a change in the size of the ovaries is noticeable, the cancer has usually spread throughout the abdominal cavity and elsewhere. Two new tests are transvaginal ultrasound, a non-invasive technique for "imaging" the ovary, and CA 125, a blood test that succeeds in about 80 percent of cases in detecting a telltale protein shed by ovarian tumors. High-risk women should get gynecological checkups at least twice a year. Some experts go so far as to urge such women, if older than 40 and finished bearing children, to consider a hysterectomy as a preventive measure. Barbara Flores knew she had the odds stacked against her. Would she be among the one in three who survived the disease?

❧ ❧ ❧

For years, she had hit the weight machines and cranked out the calisthenics at Elaine Powers. That's how she had melted her weight from 149 pounds to 125 and firmed her physique to a tensile muscularity. One morning in 1977, though, she went to her job as secretary in the library at the Norwood Elementary School, looked at the circular driveway in back and thought, Why should I pay to stay in shape? I can run right here. She wanted to keep off those extra 24 pounds, keep looking younger than her 41 years.

So she ran around the driveway every day after work, and each day she ran farther. Around and around she went, until she could complete 10 circuits, equal to about half a mile. She wanted so much to run she would have run anywhere, but the driveway was adequate. If it rained, she just asked the school custodian to let her run in the gym.

One day, she decided to try the quarter-mile track at nearby Comsewogue High School. First she ran a mile, then the next week she expanded her run to two miles, then three, and so on, each week adding a mile. She ran every day without fail. "The running was all I needed," she said. "I loved the feeling it gave me. The more I did, the more I wanted to do." The routine was simple. Barbara went home after work, changed into running clothes, headed to the track and ran. It became a central element in her life, as habitual as eating and sleeping. It never felt like a big deal, as if she had committed herself to some transcendental quest. She took it one day at a time and never planned to enter races. Within only three months, she was covering five miles on each outing. Soon all her friends and colleagues knew she was running. Hey, they wondered, what's with Barb? Ken, a former lifeguard, wondered, too. "My husband would usually think I was gone training for an awfully long time," she said. Once, nervous she was taking too long coming home from her run, Ken sent daughter Cindy to the track. "See what's taking her so long," he told her. When Cindy reached the track, Barbara said, "Tell your father I'm doing five miles today—that's what's taking me so long."

One day a friend suggested she enter a 10-kilometer race, in a shopping mall of all places. She did and placed second in the 40 to 49 age group, discovering, to her surprise, that she liked racing. It was no longer just her on the track, everything so quiet she could hear her own footsteps. It was her along with other runners, her against others, entered into a contract of competition.

Smitten by the sport, she began to compete in races every Saturday or Sunday, usually either a five or 10-kilometer, and joined a club for runners. Ken went to all her races to cheer her on, and would leave in the morning to drive to the race site and get home in the afternoon, even though the pastime ate into the weekends, especially in the summer months, when they typically went out on the "Summer Girl."

Within a few years, she compiled a streak of victories in the 40- to 49-year-old age group, remarkable for a newcomer. First in the 1981 Mistletoe Mile. First in the 1982 Smithtown Second Sight five-mile run. Second in the 1982 Bayshore Half Marathon (averaging a brisk seven minutes, 28 seconds per mile). She ran primarily to finish the races and log a respectable time. But as she came to consistently place in these events and tote home trophies, merely finishing no longer seemed enough for her. The prospective bonus of a statue, plaque, medal, or certificate fueled her with fresh incentive. Hooked now, she started to feel competitive. Wanting to win, she found herself at the starting line before a race, sizing up opponents in her age group.

Ken grew so confident about her performances that he always took victory for granted. When Barbara came home from a race, he would ask, "Oh, what award did you bring home today?" She would play a game of cat and mouse and say, "Nothing today." "Where is it?" he would kid her. Slyly, she would say, "I have no award." And he would say, "Come on now, you always bring home something." Then slowly, for dramatic effect, she would unveil her spoils for display.

Ready to turn it up a notch, she decided to train for a marathon, and on weekends she regularly ran 20 miles. In May 1982, she ran her first marathon, the *Newsday* Long Island Marathon. Few novices break four hours in a marathon. Yet she posted a time of

3:44:47, averaging about eight-and-a-half minutes a mile, for third place in the 45 to 49 age group, an outstanding performance for a first-time, 46-year-old female marathoner who had taken up running only five years earlier.

On she ran, concentrating on middle-distance races, including half-marathons. A year later she competed again in the *Newsday* event and finished in 3:46:04. In November 1988, at age 52, she completed the heralded New York City Marathon. In only a few years, she had collected several dozen awards, not to mention a jacket and, for good measure, a watch. She propped her trophies along the stairs leading to the second floor of the house, symbolic of her climb to athletic success. Little did she realize that only five months later, she would be involuntarily recruited for a race against cancer.

❦ ❦ ❦

The day after the verdict from Dr. Bruhn, Barbara ran three miles at the high-school track. She had run almost daily for 12 years. Why should she stop now? Besides, the running might be all she had. It might even ease her woes. She recalled, "I just said to myself, What's it going to matter now? I was so mixed up. I had this feeling that maybe running would straighten me out a little."

The next day she ran, too, and also the day after. As she racked up the miles, she thought, How is this going to turn out? What's going to happen to me?

"I tried to avoid thinking about my cancer as much as I could," she said. "If I thought about it, it would be too scary. Running helped keep me busy and gave me a healthier attitude. I knew very little about cancer, any kind of cancer. I never even read up on it. It was better that I had no idea. I think my ignorance about cancer was in my favor. If I had done some research, I might have driven myself nuts."

In effect, she transfused herself with regular doses of denial and even delusion. She tried to tell herself little white lies, played little games with herself. Sometimes the less one understands, the better one copes. So she tried to screen out the truth. But sustaining the falsehood proved impossible for her. She was going to die. She knew it. Just knew it, and saw no sense in fooling herself anymore. She could run all she wanted, and still this cancer in her ovaries would kill her.

Ken could no longer leave Barbara home by herself. The diagnosis had gotten her down, about as low as he had ever seen her, and not only damnably depressed but also resigned to an early grave. He decided someone should stay with her. Him, of course. He told his boss that his wife was going in for surgery and he needed to take off the next week. His boss, whose wife had recently died from a degenerative disease readily gave his consent.

❧ ❧ ❧

Ken had first spotted Barbara ice skating on a pond in Long Island with her girlfriends in 1949. He was 15, she 13. Soon after, he took her on a date to the movies but forgot to bring his money and had to call his mother for emergency funding. His first impression of Barbara was of a "full-of-fun person, terrific to be around." She had noticed Ken and found him "cute and sporty, real clean-cut and good-looking, with those dark, almond-shaped eyes." They courted and married in April 1956, and immediately set out for Washington, D.C., where he was stationed in the Navy. Two years later, they bought a four-bedroom house on Long Island, and Ken got a job at Grumman, running flight tests of F-14s and other defense aircraft.

Decade after decade, they had never lost affection for one another, and it showed. He always remembered her birthday and, of course, the big anniversary. In public, they held hands, or he put his arm around her shoulders, and sometimes he gave her a kiss for no reason other than that he loved her and wanted to remind her so. "I could search the whole world over," she said, "and never find a duplicate for him." They liked to take long walks, down Fifth Avenue in winter, along the beach in summer, and to steer "Summer Girl" toward Montauk and fish for flounder or whatever happened to be running. But just being together was enough.

And so it was now, in the heart of this deepening crisis. Ken stayed with Barbara the whole week as she awaited surgery, to divert her thoughts from the cancer. They took long walks at the beach, rode around in the car. If she wanted, they talked—about the children, about the cancer. If not, they kept quiet. He drove her all over the island in the CRX, and they admired the waterfront homes. "He never left me alone for a second," she said. But his company merely muffled her dread and melancholy.

One day, her close friend Pat Augier went over to her house to model some new running tights for her, just to goad her into a smile. But the plan backfired. Barbara, certain she would never get a chance to wear sexy tights like that, felt awful. With only two days left until surgery, Barbara said to Pat, "I'm not going to go to the hospital."

"You're going," Pat said.

"I'm not," she insisted. "I'll give you all my running clothes to wear after I'm dead."

"Do you think I'm going to listen to this?" Pat asked. "I'm not interested in inheriting your running clothes! I want my running buddy next to me on the track—in her own running clothes. You're going, and that's that."

"All right," Barbara relented. "I'm going."

The whole week, Ken kept promising Barbara the future. She would be okay, he told her. Everything would work out fine. They would get through this. Sometimes he got through to her, sometimes not. "You're healthy," he whispered in her ear. "You've got everything going for you."

Years earlier, when Barbara discovered a suspect lump under her arm, Ken had assured her it would turn out all right, and it had. In the event of trouble—any trouble—he had always told her everything would turn out all right, and it always had. Slowly she started to come around, started to believe that if she just went in for the surgery, she would come out okay. Little by little it happened, this change of mind. One day, Ken suddenly noticed the turnaround, noticed he had made her a believer.

He was driving her through town when she yelled, "Stop! Over there! I want you to take me to that store." She pointed to the shop where Pat had bought her running tights. Barbara wanted the same pair. Into the store she went, and minutes later, out she came, the owner of identical tights, black tights with turquoise stripes running down one leg, hot pink down the other. An act of optimism, this purchase, a sign of a switch in attitude. "I was starting to get aggressive about this," she recalled. "I just wanted to keep living, and I said to myself I could do it. It was just something inside of me that made me feel like that."

Now Barbara felt ready to tell her children what was going on. She told her son Kevin, a manager for the Marriott Corporation, about her condition and the upcoming operation. She invited her daughter Cindy, a sculptor and triathlete, for a walk on Cedar Beach in Mount Sinai. Cindy noticed that her mother had recently become distant and woebegone.

"Cindy, I have something to tell you," Barbara said. As they strolled, waves slapped the shore, gulls chattered, and sand crunched underfoot.

"What, Mom?"

"I have cancer." Getting right down to it.

"Oh, Mom... Oh, Mom... *No.*" Cindy stared at her mother and Barbara looked back at her. Then Cindy pressed her head against her shoulder and hugged her. "It'll be okay," Barbara said. "I'll be fine... Everything will work out." She repeated to her daughter the very words Ken had whispered to her all along. "I have something wrong with me," Barbara said now. "But I want to be here... I want to be here with you and your brother and your father... I just want you to know I'm not going to die... I'm going to live."

❦ ❦ ❦

On Monday, April 3, Barbara entered St. Charles Hospital in Port Jefferson. First Dr. Bruhn performed an exploratory laparotomy to check whether the tumors had spread. Then, over the next two hours, he performed an oophorectomy and a hysterectomy. In this procedure, he opened her stomach and removed both her ovaries, her fallopian tubes, her uterus, and her cervix.

On awakening from anesthesia, Barbara glanced over at her night table, where she had placed a photo showing her with Caryle Bethel, her New York Marathon partner. Every morning thereafter, she looked at the photo. The first time Pat visited Barbara in the room, she insisted on clipping earrings on her. Pat wanted to revive, if only symbolically, her diminished sense of normalcy and femininity.

Barbara quickly grew impatient with hospital life. "After the surgery, I had a completely different outlook, thanks to my husband and Pat," she said. "I constantly went up and down the halls. That's all I ever did. I just wanted to get moving again." Five days later, she left the hospital, and, on her first afternoon home, she went for a long walk around her neighborhood. The following morning, she attended mass.

Soon after her arrival home, Barbara visited oncologist Dr. Harish Malhotra. Gently he told her that her biopsy had come back negative—no evidence of spread throughout the lymphatic system—but with a caveat. A tumor marker called CA 125 indicated a high probability of recurrence. Malhotra recommended chemotherapy as a precaution, the better to avert another surgery down the road. He explained that starting immediately she would need to receive massive doses of cytoxin and cisplatin, in intravenous injections every three or four weeks, for the next eight months. He warned her of severe side effects, from nausea, vomiting, and hair loss to extreme fatigue, weakness, and a drop in blood count.

"It's a difficult period for patients and there are no guarantees," Malhotra said. "We let Barbara know we were with her and would try to make it as easy as we could. We'd hold her hand and walk her through it. Some patients take comfort and reassurance in this. The typical reaction, however, is a mixture of anxiety, fear, anger, sadness, and withdrawal. The news is depressing, and starts to sink in. Most patients will ask, 'Are you trying to tell me you're going to make me sick to make me better?'"

"But Barbara appeared to be a go-getter," he said. "She quickly got in control of her situation and decided to deal with it. It was easy to work with her. She always had a smile on her face. Her attitude appeared to be, Go ahead and do whatever you have to do, I'm going to lick it and live a normal life."

Each chemo session in the hospital was scheduled to take two days. For the first session, Barbara stayed three days and four nights. Afterward, she felt so drained that she needed to take a day or so to bounce back. She took even longer to rebound after the second visit, and realized the next time would be worse. She thought, This is too much. This is taking too much out of me. No more. "I hated going to the hospital for chemo," she said. "I felt like a prisoner being all hooked up."

Besides, she and Ken disliked being apart overnight. She wanted to go in for chemo early in the morning and be back at home—in her own bed, with her husband of three decades—the same night. Barbara told Dr. Malhotra of her strong preference to be an outpatient. Permission granted, she went to her third chemo session at St. Charles Hospital at five in the morning and wrapped it all up by five in the afternoon. "It's most uncharacteristic for a patient to go through this heavy a regimen in so short a time," Malhotra said, "But Barbara had made up her mind."

The outpatient idea was no cure-all, just an abbreviation of a punishing process, and Barbara still fell prey to the side effects of chemo. She was nauseated and her stomach hurt. She lost her appetite and vomited again and again. The whole works, except for the shedding of hair. Her hair stayed on her scalp, but turned an attractive platinum blonde.

She and Ken took long walks at the beach at every opportunity. Looking long and lean, she might wear white shorts, a blue tank top, matching skirt and dangling earrings—an athlete still. She envisioned herself finishing chemo and walking out of the hospital for the last time. Such mental rehearsal for reality, she found, was like controlling a dream. She imagined how this scenario would play out in enough detail to program herself for the event itself. The idea was that if she could picture herself surviving this disease, the odds automatically increased that she would.

Ken stayed with Barbara as long and as often as he could, at home and in the hospital. He wanted to cater to her, to prepare her dinner, to handle housework. He tiptoed around her at home, offering to do this or that. Was she comfortable? Could he get her some yogurt or something? Did she mind if he put on the TV? Would she like to lie down? It got to be a bit annoying after awhile, well-intentioned as her husband was, and Barbara would have none of it. "Sympathy is no good for me," she said. "I dislike being babied. I could eat nothing, I could drink nothing, and he could do nothing to make me feel any better."

She sensed his frustration at being unable to help her and, for his sake, asked him to leave, to just go away. Now, after the sixth chemo session, Barbara desperately wanted to quit the treatments, and told Pat so. "I'm going to give you all my running clothes," Barbara said, "because I'm going to die." She acted like Camille doing her deathbed scene. But Pat refused to buy the act.

"No, you're not," her friend said. "You better get your treatments. You better do what I tell you. I'm going to stay here until you change your mind. I'm going to stay here until you're sick of seeing me and hearing my voice."

Pat stayed with Barbara for three hours that day, alternately giving her a pep talk and chewing her out. "She saw me vomiting and suffering," Barbara recalled. "But she stared me right in the face and gave me no sympathy, and I liked that. I needed that."

Meanwhile, only a month after surgery, she wanted to return to running. She had vegetated long enough. Now she wanted that special lift that only running could give her, the boost that enabled her to feel alive again. Bruhn and Malhotra encouraged her to run, but also cautioned her against too much too soon.

"I told her to try not to push it too much," said Dr. Bruhn, who himself lifts weights, rides a bicycle, and climbs a Stairmaster at least three times a week. "It was okay with me as long as she took it easy. I warned her that she better lay off the marathons for awhile. I was worried that if she ran too soon after surgery, she might overextend herself and get a hernia from the incision."

"I told her that if she could move, she should," Dr. Malhotra said. "Any form of muscular activity is beneficial, because cisplatin chemo weakens the muscles and nerves. But I worried that her running would cause extreme fatigue. Still, she decided she was going to put up with it. So I said to her, 'Okay, keep doing what you're doing.'"

Recalled Barbara, "I knew the doctors were going to tell me I could run—I already had my running clothes on. I felt from the beginning that because of my running, I would be a stronger person. Even the nurses told me, 'If you stay in good shape, you'll tolerate the chemo better.'"

During treatment she taped the following Hallmark poster on her wall at home:

"Why do I run,
t'ain't no mystery,
wanna have a good medical history,
Doctor told me running is great,
helps them blood cells circulate,
great for the lungs, great for the ticker,
can't nothing get you in better shape quicker,
feels so healthy, feels so sweet,
pumping my arms and flapping my feet.
Moving my muscles, firming my form,
panting like a pack mule, sweating up a storm,
keeps me youthful, keeps me loose,
tightens my tummy and shrinks my caboose,
beats being sluggish, beats being lazy,
why do I run, maybe I'm crazy."

Within a few months, through subsequent chemo sessions, Barbara was running hard, logging as many as seven or eight miles a day, sometimes even covering more miles than she had before the diagnosis. And seven months after her surgery, she completed the New York City Marathon. She walked the whole distance, at a rate of about 13 minutes per mile, and finished in 5:48:23.

"It was really something to see," Ken said. "Her plugging away, going the whole distance. And so soon after her operation. While still going through chemo."

Malhotra, who has run half-marathons, said, "I know what it takes to do a marathon. That's a lot of effort, especially for a chemo patient—and all the more so for one no longer in the prime of her youth. I was totally shocked."

Two weeks after the marathon, Barbara finished her last cycle of chemo.

❣ ❣ ❣

Barbara ran in dozens of races over the next three years, always placing in the 50–59 category, sometimes finishing first. First in the 5K West Meadow Beach Sprint. First in the 1992 Village Way Annual Run. First in the Fifth Annual St. James 5-Mile Striding

Event. First in the 1992 Park Bench 5K. Still improving, she shaved eight minutes off her time for the Long Island Half Marathon, from 2:18 in 1991 to 2:11 in 1992. Most important, she bucked the odds, becoming among the lucky one in three victims of ovarian cancer to go into remission.

"A lot of cancer patients refuse to accept the diagnosis," Dr. Bruhn observed. "They keep going around getting other opinions and canceling surgery. If they think they're going to die, they lay down and die. But Barbara and I knew each other and she trusted me. She was intelligent enough to realize that she had no choice but surgery and chemo, and that was the bottom line.

"I think she is probably special, and that her success against ovarian cancer is partly due to her outlook, her positive attitude. I have only a few patients like her. She wanted to get back to running, to competing, as soon as she could, and it would not surprise me if her running helped her get better. With that combination of athleticism and desire, it probably did. She had an edge because something inside her told her not to give up, and she was matter-of-fact that she was going to beat it. Cancer was another hurdle in life for her to get over."

Dr. Malhotra concurred: "She is unusual, no question about it. Most people dwell on the cancer, look for sympathy, say, 'Oh God, I've gone through hell, I can hardly move.' Barbara was not like that. She said to herself, 'Hey, I've got to go do this marathon and I'm going to do it, no matter what anyone says.' Not everybody is able to do that. She's provided us all with a lesson that you can control a lot with your attitude and concentration.

"Certainly physical exercise and athletics raise your threshold of pain and your ability to deal with depression, but I attribute it to pure force of will. I've practiced for 12 years and seen thousands of patients—in fact, I saw 70 only today—and I've never seen a patient like her. She actually completed a marathon during chemotherapy. Most *healthy* people cannot run marathons. For her to do that, God bless her. I just wish more patients were like her. Absolutely. I must have told her that a million times."

Now 56, Barbara is back at her job. She goes for general checkups with Dr. Malhotra every three months and annually for mammography and CAT scans. On the anniversary of her surgery, Ken always hands her a dozen red roses. And still she runs, mostly in five and 10-kilometer races and half-marathons.

"I still have a special feeling from running," she said. "Sure, some days you start out stiff and you suffer. But then you go a mile and you feel this euphoria. It's a feeling that nothing else matters. Your mind is free and clear, and you believe you can achieve anything."

"Running is so rewarding," she said, "but now I want to bring down my times. Why not? I mean, I'm happy with my all my plaques and trophies. But I want more."

Chapter 3

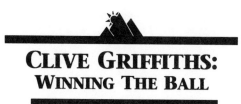

CLIVE GRIFFITHS:
WINNING THE BALL

Rude as it seems, especially given his audience of teenage boys, Clive Griffiths, the former professional soccer player, is talking testicles.

"Someone tell me," he says to the several hundred high school boys assembled in an auditorium. "Tell me what your nuts feel like." Titters and giggles break out. No one answers. Griffiths again asks the question, but nobody puts up his hand.

"Peanuts," says a voice from the back. Chuckles all around.

Clive smiles a 250-watt smile at the podium, brushes back his thick, black, curly hair and laughs. "Always a smart aleck, wherever I go.

"Well, boys," he continues, "the point is this: most of you have no idea what they really feel like. But you should, because, as you will agree, testicles are important. Hit me anywhere but in the nuts, right? If you have a problem with your testicles, how are you going to tell, unless you know what they feel like in a normal state? Now, if you twist your ankle, you can go to your mom and say, 'Hey, Mom, check my ankle out.' But your testicles are a different story. 'Hey, Mom, check my nuts out.' It would be embarrassing for you to do. So *you've* got to know what they feel like."

Griffiths is a volunteer spokesman for the American Cancer Society. His mission is to promote awareness and increase detection of cancer of the testicles. He's spoken at hundreds of high schools and junior highs all across the state of Kansas, as well as in Missouri and California. He gives talks to kids aged anywhere from 13 to 18, usually in an auditorium or gymnasium or sometimes a classroom, addressing as few as 15 students or as many as 900.

To begin, Griffiths shows a 15-minute videotape he helped develop with the University of Iowa hospitals and clinics. In the film, Clive dashes around the soccer field, his hair flopping. He leaps to block a kick, passes off for a goal, hugs a teammate, and raises a fist in exultation. Then, the film over, he approaches the microphone.

"I was an athlete, 28 years old, in the prime of my career," he quietly tells the audience. "My career was a roller coaster I thought would never end. In the film you just saw, here's this happy guy, playing with a team that sells out every game, a real success story. And then—boom!—cancer. No one would have thought I was a candidate for cancer. But it can strike anyone. At any time."

The audience falls into a hush. "The last thought on my mind," says Griffiths, "was getting cancer." Then Griffiths briefly describes his diagnosis, treatment, and recovery. No more giggles now, just throats clearing, bodies shifting in seats. His message is that they, too, can get this disease—and that if they do, they can survive it. The theme, however, is early detection through education. He underscores the importance of boys regularly examining themselves for lumps and other abnormalities. "It can save, if not your life, then some of the pain and heartache of agonizing treatments," Griffiths says. "If I had known then what I know now, I could have saved myself from radical surgery and chemotherapy."

In closing, he fields questions from students and passes out a brochure about testicular self-examination and a reminder card for boys to place in the shower.

"I never want to sound like a professor coming out with big, technical words," Griffiths said after the talk. "They'll just fall asleep without learning anything. Obviously, to young boys, the subject of testicles is sometimes going to seem hysterically funny. I use different terms—family jewels, nuts, balls, goolies, danglers, whatever—and I get the kids rolling in the aisles. But I want kids to be familiar with this danger so they can diagnose it early and keep the percentages in favor of survival. My message is that early detection and self-examination are the best protection. You should never mess around with testicular cancer.

"Believe me. I know."

❦ ❦ ❦

Clive Griffiths started playing organized soccer at 11 years of age for his local YMCA team in South Wales. A teenage boy came knocking at his door one day and said, "Listen, we're short a man and you're big enough to play for us. Will you come help us out with a game we've got today?" Griffiths told the boy he had no soccer shoes. So the kid borrowed a pair of soccer shoes from a friend of his down the street, and Clive wore those shoes in his first soccer game. He played well, well enough to be invited back for another game, and then another. Soon he had established himself as a formidable presence on the local YMCA team. The men from the neighborhood encouraged the boy to compete in games ordinarily reserved only for adults.

Clive lived in a small town called Pontypridd, in South Wales. It was a mountainous place, a coal-mining community. The coal miners rode the elevators down into the shafts (in those days without the benefit of masks protecting against black lung disease) and mined that coal from the bowels of purgatory. Clive would start delivering newspapers at 5:30 a.m. and spot the workers shambling home from the mines. "Those poor old geezers always panted and puffed from all the dust they had inhaled, dragging themselves home at sunrise," Clive recalled. "Most of the kids who came out of school in Pontypridd went to work in those coal mines. My parents would say, 'You better finish your homework and do well in school or else you'll end up in those mines.'"

Clive had always excelled as an all-around athlete. At age 14, he was already nearly fully grown, a rugged and energetic 5 feet, 9 inches and 160 pounds. In school, he ran the fastest sprints and hurdles, jumped the farthest long jump, outdistanced all comers in cross-country races, even won consistently in ping-pong and snooker. Soccer came naturally. "When I started playing soccer, it was no big deal," he said. "What do you want me to do?" he would ask the coach. "Kick the ball? Just tell me where to kick it."

Clive's soccer prowess kept him out of the mines. The Manchester United soccer team offered him a contract, and Manchester United was no ordinary soccer team; it was the most popular, most powerful soccer club in Europe—the New York Yankees of English, first-division soccer. For Clive, Manchester United was *the* team. "I lived and breathed Manchester United. When a chance came to sign a contract, I jumped all over it."

He stayed in school for a year, commuting about 250 miles for games. At 15, he dropped out of school and moved to England—away from his family—to start with the team as an apprentice professional, the equivalent of a U.S. minor-league baseball player. He earned $15 a week, plus room and board, and lived with a family in Manchester.

Griffiths rose fast through the ranks and reached the Manchester reserves by 16. At age 18, a full-time professional living on his own, he joined the first team and played with the top pros in the land. He rode the first-division circuit, from Birmingham and Sheffield to Liverpool and London, and played in front of vast,

raucous crowds of 40,000 to 50,000, going head-to-head against
the best players in Europe, if not the world.

By happenstance, his youth coach at Manchester United
became head coach for the Chicago Sting of the North American
Soccer League (NASL), a national organization with franchises
from coast to coast, including New York and Los Angeles. The
coach quickly invited Griffiths to play for him. In 1975, Griffiths
hopped a plane for Chicago. The Welsh lad was coming to the
United States. He was 19 years old.

❦ ❦ ❦

If Griffiths had a specialty in soccer, even as a youngster on
the local YMCA team, it was defense. He left the glamour and
glory to the scorers. From the start with Manchester United, he
had made his name as a defender. He would keep vigil in the
middle, a kamikaze doing all the dirty work. He played on the
back line, usually as a defensive end, sometimes as a central
halfback or right fullback. There, in a midfield zone he appropriated
as his personal property, Griffiths anchored the defense for his
team. Goalkeepers loved him. Any player who had the misfortune
to be in possession of the ball while daring to trespass on his
territory was deserving of pity. He had no letup in him at all.
With his speed, Clive could keep pace with almost anyone in any
league. In his zeal, he clearly lived to deny success to the other side.

Griffiths always set his sights on guarding the best forward,
the most prolific scorer, on the opposing team, and usually pulled
such an assignment anyway. His coach would say, "OK, Clive,
there's the best player, off you go now. Take care of him." He
seldom waited for an opponent to make his move; rather, he
would anticipate the direction in which the adversary might
dribble or pass or butt the ball, then position himself for a well-
timed charge to the ball. Search and destroy, that's how he
operated. He lit out after cross-field passes, stayed on the heels of
opponents, barged in to break up plays. He swiped the dribble
and chipped passes upfield to scorers and swung his team into a
group of attackers. Once, Griffiths went man-to-man against the
legendary Brazilian, Pelé himself.

If Griffiths had a trademark, it was the slide tackle. He would
barrel toward an opponent and, starting about five feet away,
slide legs first, his legs slicing like a pair of scissors, bring down
the player and retrieve the ball for his team. If you thought of
Clive, you thought of the slide tackle. But he had a technique
that gave the move an extra dimension. While most defenders

who performed slide tackles would simply knock the ball out of play, enabling the other team to regain possession of it, Griffiths would clamp his foot onto the top of the ball and bounce from the field into a standing position, all in one fell swoop, with his feet ready to pass the ball to a teammate.

There went the black-and-white checkered ball down the field, sailing through the air, skidding across the grass. And there went Clive Griffiths after it. An opponent would gather in the ball and start to dribble downfield on a breakaway, looking to deliver a pass to an open teammate. And Griffiths would bird-dog the ballhandler without mercy, latching onto the heels of his cleats like a pit bull after its prey. The adversary would rear back his right leg and swing into a hard thud of a kick, sending the ball spinning and curving high toward the front of the goal. And Griffiths would backpedal furiously, a tape suddenly shifted into rewind, and follow the shot as it twisted lower and lower toward the goalie, a score in the making. Clive would then take flight, all 5 feet, 10 inches of him, a kangaroo on a trampoline, soaring over players taller than he, and bop the shot away with his head, killing the threat to his team.

He played hurt, rarely complained, and seldom missed a game despite pulled hamstrings, torn ligaments, and other injuries. The Sting played on Astroturf, and Clive—what with his helter-skelter gallops downfield, his dives and his slide tackles—would return to the locker room with his legs all chewed up from the artificial turf, riddled with bloody, pus-filled scratches known as "strawberries." One time an opposing player elbowed him in the thick of a tussle over the ball and broke his nose. But the trainers and managers had no clue until the game was over that Clive was even in the least bit hurt. The Chicago sportswriters nicknamed him the "Iron Man." Such durability would soon come in handy.

❦ ❦ ❦

He met Marylee Swain, an attractive, blond kindergarten teacher, backstage at a Chicago public television station in 1978. Several days later, Marylee impetuously wrote him a rather unorthodox fan letter. "If you're married," she wrote, "throw this letter away and kiss your wife. If not, call me." Clive called, and in June 1979, they married.

Four months later, he was traded to the Tulsa Roughnecks, an NASL franchise in Oklahoma. As had happened in England and Chicago, so it went in Tulsa. Griffiths—with a rock-star mane an inch from his shoulders and his high-voltage charisma—quickly became a fan favorite, a hero to males, a heartthrob to females. Nevertheless, a year later he was shipped out again, back to Chicago, only this time to play for the Chicago Horizons in a different organization, the Major Indoor Soccer League (MISL). But after a single season, the team folded. Fortunately for Griffiths, the coach, Luis Dabo, took the helm for the Kansas City Comets, also of the indoor league, and in 1981 he recruited Griffiths, the defensive impresario, to play for him again. When Griffiths landed at Kansas City International Airport, he officially ended his days as a soccer gypsy.

The Comets, formerly the San Francisco Fog, were a new franchise, hungry for publicity and brand-name attractions. Griffiths would captain the team, as he had the Sting, the Roughnecks, and the Horizons, leading not by bellowing pep talks but by setting the right example for teammates to follow. Two months into the season, the Comets fired Dabo and hired a new coach, Pat McBride. In Griffiths' first season in Kansas City, the Comets fared poorly, posting a 14–30 record.

Still, it was a winning time for Griffiths. He was sworn in as a U.S. citizen. One December morning, at the Federal Building in downtown Kansas City, he recited the Pledge of Allegiance and took an oath renouncing his previous citizenship. After the naturalization ceremony, Clive, in a three-piece pinstriped suit, waved a small American flag for newspaper photographers. He said, "Probably all the good in my life has come from the United States—a good career, a good family, good surroundings, good friends." Marylee joked that she would no longer have to worry about his losing his green card.

Clive quickly gained the same popularity he had had on his previous teams. He became involved with many charitable organizations, including the Ronald McDonald House program, the Leukemia Society, and the Kansas and Missouri Special Olympics. But none of his pro bono commitments touched him more than the case of Casey Regan, a pudgy 11-year-old girl with braces and pimples who played soccer and attended Comets games. Her parents called the Comets one day because Casey had leukemia, and they wanted to know whether a player from the club could visit her in the hospital and possibly autograph a soccer ball for her, just to raise her spirits.

So Clive visited Casey, not once or twice but several times, both at the hospital and, later, at her home. On his first visit, he went alone, minus newspaper photographers but bearing free merchandise. He handed her a Comets T-shirt, a wristband, a cap, a team poster and an autographed sweatshirt. They shared some cookies and tea. Two days before Christmas, her mother, Jan, wrote Clive a letter: "You have a heart made of gold! It was so great of you to come by and visit with Casey and her friends.... Our many thanks to you for sharing your time and darling personality with us. You really made a very sick little girl very happy!"

Clive's concern for Casey Regan would someday yield dividends many times over.

❦ ❦ ❦

In March 1983, Griffiths, now 28, was playing at the height of his ability. In only 33 games, he had already blocked 71 shots, the second-best defensive record in the Major Indoor Soccer League. He had also become more offense-minded, with a goal and eight assists. He competed in the same style as before, never fiddled with the formula, played to his strengths. The Kansas City Comets had a 19–14 record, and at one point, won 14 of 16 games.

The team was on the road, playing back-to-back games in California, against the San Jose Earthquakes and the San Diego Sockers. Griffiths played well, and the team won both games. The club arrived home on a Saturday. Griffiths remembers the circumstances because the events foretold a new chapter in his life.

"On Saturday evening I was in bed with Marylee," he said. "And she touched me down there. I jumped up and screamed. It was on the right side of my testicle. Very tender and painful. A heavy feeling in the scrotum. And I said to her, 'Don't do that!' Marylee said, 'What's the matter? That's the first time I ever heard you complain about that.' It felt like a bulge or a swelling in my groin. So we figured something was wrong. I decided to go get myself checked out." On Monday, March 8, Griffiths had an appointment with Dr. Karl Kurtz, a urologist at the Suburban Medical Center. The next day, he returned for a second exam. Clive underwent several diagnostic tests, including an X-ray, an alpha-fetoprotein count, an ultrasound, and a sonogram. As it happened, back in 1968, Dr. Kurtz had seen a man with similar symptoms. But the physician had abruptly ruled out the likelihood of testicular cancer, and the patient had later developed the disease, and, as a direct consequence, died. Suspecting testicular cancer in Griffiths, and determined to avoid a fatal oversight, Kurtz twice checked the soccer player, just to clear his conscience. Then, he sent him home, promising to let him know the test results the next day.

The following morning, Griffiths attended an 11:00 a.m. kick-around with his team. During the practice session, Kurtz left a message on his telephone answering machine. Griffiths, on hearing the tape, immediately called Kurtz back.

"Clive," Kurtz said, "the sonogram confirmed what I suspected. The tests show a tumor. You'd better come in this afternoon for a talk."

"Okay, fine," Griffiths said, "but I have a game tonight. How about if I just play tonight?"

Griffiths had had a vague premonition about scoring his second goal of the season that night. Besides, the Comets were hurtling toward the league playoffs. Reflexively, he wanted to shrug off the diagnosis of a tumor in his testicle as just another obstacle to be overcome, no different, really, from a pulled hamstring or a torn ligament. He'd played soccer almost half his life, competing in mud and rain against the roughest of the rough. "I'd had injuries before and gone on to play again," Griffiths recalled. "I had an easy, free-spirit attitude toward injuries. In talking with the doctor, I figured, After the game tomorrow I'll be all yours, and we'll learn some more about this tumor in my groin. I'm thinking, No big deal, it'll go away. I'm thinking, Hey, it's only a cancer of the testicles. They'll take out the tumor, end of story."

Before his happy-go-lucky thoughts could gain momentum, Kurtz answered, "Absolutely not."

"Why not?" After all, Griffiths was the Iron Man.

"Clive, listen to me," the urologist said. "You have a tumor. If you play in the game tonight and you take a hard kick in the groin, or the ball strikes you in that spot—it would take just one shot—it could split the tumor. If the tumor splits, the cancer could go out of control and spread all over your body. You could get in trouble. You could die."

Tell me something else, Clive thought. Tell me I've torn a ligament. Tell me I've broken my leg. But not cancer. We're fighting for the playoffs.

"You need to understand," Kurtz said. "We're talking life and death."

That afternoon, Griffiths went to Kurtz's office. The physician explained that, although testicular cancer is among the fastest-growing of all cancers, it is also among the most curable—if arrested in time.

God, this is no joking matter, Griffiths thought. "Okay," he said, "let's do what we have to do."

"We have to operate on Thursday," Kurtz said.

"Thursday? That's rather quick. Whatever it is, can we hold off on surgery until the end of the season?"

"You'll probably have to sit out the rest of the season." Kurtz would have to perform an orchiectomy—removal of the testicle. Then he would have to conduct a biopsy and peer through a microscope to study the tissue taken out and assess the kind of tumor involved. He sketched a drawing approximating the surgery. It would require a sliver of an incision, like the cut for an appendectomy, in the wall of the abdomen. He would then pinch the scrotum to pop the testicle—and the suspicious mass growing inside it—through a canal, into the abdomen, and remove it through the groin.

Most men who undergo this operation, Kurtz pointed out, retain the ability for erection and orgasm, and continue to be sexually active and fertile. But he would render no judgment about any treatment that might be necessary after the orchiectomy, nor speculate on Clive's prognosis for recovery—at least not until the biopsy revealed which of the four kinds of tumor Griffiths had and to what extent it might have spread.

❦ ❦ ❦

Clive had to tell Marylee. Just one hitch: Marylee was pregnant, more than 7 months along. Three years earlier, at the age of 27, she had miscarried. After 12 weeks of pregnancy, she had hemorrhaged. An ambulance had rushed her to a hospital, where physicians discovered that the fetus inside her had stopped growing after three weeks and died. For a year after the miscarriage, Marylee had struggled to decide whether to try again. And for 18 months the Griffiths had tried to conceive another child.

Now Marylee was again pregnant, and the baby was expected in about six weeks. Clive thought, I might not even be here to see my first child.

After the visit to Dr. Kurtz, Clive called his wife at her job. "Marylee," he said, softly and slowly. "Dr. Kurtz is 85 percent sure the tumor is cancerous. He needs to go in and take a look."

Marylee thought: Cancer equals death. I have to be with him. She hung up the telephone and shouted to her boss that she had to leave immediately. She rushed to her car, sobbing, and pulled onto Interstate 35. She gunned the car down the expressway, glancing at the speedometer. Soon she found herself racing at 95 miles per hour. "I was in such shock," Marylee recalled. "I was in a panic, and I wanted to get home to my husband. I needed to be there for him physically. It was as if I thought I could get between Clive and the tumor."

Marylee reached the house, flung open the door, and embraced her husband. Then she began to cry.

Later that afternoon, Clive went to Kemper Arena, where the Comets played, to the office of Pat McBride. He told the coach that he would have to skip the game that night. "Well, what's the problem?" McBride asked.

"We're probably talking cancer here."

McBride had no idea what to say.

That night the Griffiths attended the Comets game against San Jose. Spectators who recognized Clive as a Comet wondered why he was out of action. The Comets won, 6–1, tying San Diego for first place in the Western Division. Afterward, McBride said, "Our thoughts were with Clive the whole game. Tonight he gave us an extra incentive. We wanted to win this one for him."

In the tension over the upcoming operation, Marylee sought to leaven the atmosphere with humor. "We decided, what the heck, it's no good being long-faced about it," Clive said. Teasing her husband, Marylee joked that after the surgery, he could park his car in spaces for the handicapped.

On Wednesday, March 10, Clive entered the Suburban Medical Center in Overland Park for the orchiectomy, scheduled for the next morning. Marylee spent the night at home alone. As she lay awake, she had grave misgivings about the tumor. What if I lose Clive? What if I have to raise our child without him?

The orchiectomy lasted about an hour. As Marylee sat in the waiting room, she embroidered a baby blanket. Dr. Kurtz took out a tumor about the size of a nickel. Now the Griffiths had to wait 48 hours for the biopsy report.

Hundreds of Comets fans sent flowers and cards to Clive at the hospital. Little kids called the center to wish him well, the switchboard patching through calls to his room. Coach McBride and teammates visited Clive, stumped about how, or whether, to broach the subject of cancer. "What do you say?" teammate Gino Schiraldi asked. "How do you act?"

The day after the surgery, McBride appointed Comets teammate Greg Makowski, a league all-star the previous season, to step into the breach as captain of the club.

Casey Regan, the sixth-grade leukemia patient Clive had visited in the hospital the previous year, now came to see him. She had sustained a series of relapses before finally going into an apparently permanent remission. Casey had gotten the idea that during his visits to her, she had given him cancer. He had to reassure her that cancer was not contagious.

The biopsy report came back from the pathologist on Saturday afternoon. Dr. Kurtz, looking somber, approached

Clive and Marylee. I'm in real trouble now, Clive thought.

"We've got bad news," Kurtz said.

"Okay, Doc, what is it?"

The couple inhaled and waited for the doctor to deliver the verdict.

"I've just come back from church, where I prayed for guidance. I prayed so I could come here to the hospital and tell you both— a young couple expecting a baby, here at what is supposed to be the happiest point in your lives—that the tumor has spread. Clive is going to need further surgery."

The biopsy, Kurtz explained, had disclosed a rare malignancy. The tumor consisted of not just one cell growth commonly found in testicular cancer, not even two—but, quite surprisingly, three. Type I testicular cancer is confined to the testicle, and an orchiectomy usually proves adequate as treatment; Type II spreads—or, in technical terms, metastasizes—upwards into the diaphragm and invades the lymphatic system, attacking the lymph nodes. Type III, most serious of all, penetrates the bloodstream. The biopsy, Kurtz went on, suggested that about 25 percent of the tumor had already fanned out into his lymphatic system. If the malignancy traveled to his internal organs, it could be deadly.

As the first order of business, Clive would need at least two weeks to heal from the orchiectomy. Then he would have to undergo another operation to remove the cancerous lymph nodes, an intricate and complex procedure called a lymphadenectomy. Kurtz answered questions and offered comfort to the Griffiths for two hours that night in the hospital.

A week later, Clive met with Dr. John Weigel, a surgeon at the University of Kansas Medical Center in Kansas City, who would perform the lymphadenectomy with Dr. Kurtz's assistance. Weigel explained that the procedure typically improved the chances of survival for a patient from about 40 percent to 60 percent. He warned that the operation could sever his sympathetic nerve, which controls ejaculation. If the nerve is cut, the patient is no longer capable of ejaculating sperm and, by extension, of inseminating a female. In other words, Griffiths ran the risk— roughly a 50-50 proposition—of becoming unable to father any more children.

As the date for the second surgery approached, the situation imposed inordinate stress on Marylee. Though well into her final trimester of pregnancy, she had lost rather than gained weight for several weeks in a row. She also had cervical complications. Her obstetrician-gynecologist, Richard Sinclair, examined Marylee daily.

Finally, Dr. Sinclair recommended that she stop working until she delivered the baby.

"I know you're concerned about Clive," Dr. Sinclair said. "But you've got to worry about yourself, too. You're all thinned out and you're going to dilate real soon. I want you to slow down and relax... We have enough problems on our hands. If you deliver early, we could have a premature baby."

❦ ❦ ❦

Cancer of the testicles annually strikes 5,500 men in the United States and, in an estimated 400 cases, leads to death. A relatively rare disease, it accounts for only about 1 percent of cancers in American men. Testicular cancer predominates in young men, those between the ages of 15 and 40, at the prime of fertility. In the last 40 years, the rate for this condition among white men has, alarmingly, nearly doubled.

The testes are suspended from the body by the spermatic cord and are enclosed in the scrotum, a pouch of membrane and loose skin. They are, of course, the male reproductive glands. They produce the spermatozoa essential to fertilize female egg cells and also generate the male hormone testosterone.

The most common symptom of testicular cancer is a hard, usually painless, lump on the testicle. A nodule, a swelling, or a sensation of heaviness or dragging in the lower abdomen or scrotum may also indicate a tumor. Diagnosis of a suspected tumor is generally confirmed by either a chest X-ray, a computerized axial tomography (CAT) scan of the pelvis and abdomen, or blood tests for telltale tumor markers such as alpha-fetoprotein. Other diagnostic tests are ultrasound—bouncing high-frequency sound waves off body tissue to yield images of the internal structures of the body—and radionuclide scans that show the presence of cancer cells.

Recent developments in treatment have made possible a complete cure for 80 percent to 90 percent of patients, even for those whose cases are advanced. Testicular cancer has one of the highest cure rates of all cancers. Anticancer drugs are progressively more potent and effective than ever. Unfortunately, many young men, though aware of an abnormality in a testis, are reluctant to see a doctor. Sometimes, they mistakenly believe that a lump may go away by itself.

The American Cancer Society recommends that young men conduct a monthly testicular self-examination (TSE). It takes only a minute or two. Ideally, this exam is done after a warm shower or bath, when the skin of the scrotum is relaxed and anything unusual can be felt. You simply stand in front of a mirror and gently roll each testis between the thumb and fingers of both hands. The testicles should be egg-shaped and feel smooth and rubbery. Check for changes in size, shape, and color. Examine the front, sides, and back of each testicle. If you find a lump, feel an ache, or sense any other change, you should contact a physician immediately.

Untreated, testicular cancer can spread through the body with sinister speed. The human body is a network of lymph nodes, and cancer can ride the byways of the lymphatic system. From the testicles, a malignant tumor can infiltrate the chest and the lungs and penetrate the bloodstream, its deadly cells capable of multiplying threefold within a month and turning up virtually anywhere in the body.

❦ ❦ ❦

On March 24, Clive went to the University of Kansas Medical Center for the lymphadenectomy. Marylee arranged for him to enter the hospital under the alias "John Smith"—even for the sign on the door to his room to say "John Smith"—to divert attention from her husband. Even so, young Comets fans spilled into the hospital lobby, swarming around the security guards.

"Where's Clive?"

"Which room is he in?"

"Can we go see him?"

The operation was expected to last five hours. Dr. Weigel cut down from the diaphragm to enter the lymph nodes. He delved in, not through the back—the approximate location of the lymph nodes—but through the front of the stomach wall, to prevent damage to the spine. In a long, tedious process—a search-and-destroy mission—the surgeon scanned the lymphatic tract with his naked eye, digging meticulously for his target: the 25 percent of renegade cancer cells still lingering in the lymph nodes.

Because Clive was an athlete, Dr. Weigel had to deal with some special difficulties, and the procedure extended to more than six hours. The surgeon had a problem keeping the incision in his stomach open wide enough to root around. Clive's abdominal muscles were so taut and well-developed that the opening kept flapping defiantly shut. Weigel also had trouble sewing up the incision. The thread woven through the skin, again because of his washboard stomach muscles, kept snapping in two.

Marylee squirmed in the waiting room, expecting a birth while frightened of the hovering specter of death. As the hours passed, she settled into a make-busy task. She addressed the envelopes containing the card that would announce the much-anticipated arrival of the newest Griffiths.

During the operation, Dr. Weigel found 11 lymph nodes, three of which were infected. All the nodes had moved rapidly through his system, one inching close to the diaphragm, directly under his chest and lungs. He extracted all 11 nodes.

Clive stayed overnight in intensive care, a zipper of a scar now spanning his body from his crotch to the middle of his sternum, and soldiered through the postoperative pain. "He never complained," Marylee recalled. "Never even asked for any pain medicine. What bothered him was lying on his back, being forced to stay inactive. He wanted to get up and run around."

After the lymphadenectomy, a second biopsy aroused new concerns about Clive's condition. The latest tissue sample hinted that fugitive cells, the vestiges of malignancy, still floated somewhere in his bloodstream. Time for another search-and-destroy mission—and for the question of chemotherapy.

As Clive recuperated, Dr. Ron Stevens, director of oncology at the hospital, came around to discuss his options for chemo. He explained the drugs that would be used, the consequences of going through treatment, and the risks of skipping it. "Only about 1 percent of the cancer cells are still inside you," Stevens explained. "You can get chemotherapy, and your chance of survival will probably be about 95 percent. Or you can do nothing and ride this out. But you should know that, without chemo, those odds drop to roughly 40 percent."

What kind of a choice is that? Clive thought. "Hey, listen," he said, "give me the drugs."

❦ ❦ ❦

A few days after Clive left the hospital, Dr. Weigel informed him that the operation had, in fact, severed the sympathetic nerve supply. He could father no more children. As soon as the Griffiths heard the news, Clive turned to Marylee and shrugged. "That's life," he said, appearing more casual than he felt. "Besides, we already have a bun in the oven."

❦ ❦ ❦

Clive's father John had earned a modest living as a machinery repairman. With his wife Muriel, he had raised seven children—five sons, two daughters, with Clive numerically in the middle—in a government housing project in Pontypridd. "Our house probably had no more square footage than the basement I have now," Clive recalled. "With seven kids around, my mom had no time to take care of everything for me and worry about my every little nick and scrape. She was always cleaning and washing. So my brothers and sisters and I just had to look after ourselves."

Self-sufficient from the beginning, Clive took a job in a grocery store at age 10. Then he added a newspaper route, waking at 5:30 a.m. to deliver 400 papers. He turned over to his family his entire weekly income of $2.50. He washed his own socks, ironed his own pants and shirts, and cooked his own dinners.

"I had only one uniform to wear for soccer three or four times a week. So I washed and ironed it myself rather than bother Mom. As kids, we were never mollycoddled. I was brought up in a community where people never looked for sympathy. They got on with life and did what they had to do." Clive got on with it, all right. As a 12-year-old playing soccer for the YMCA, he had gastric flu a few days before a Saturday game. He vomited copiously, ran a fever, and had difficulty straightening out his back. But he went out and played, the spectators noticing he was sweating and flushed and red-faced. Still, he never told anyone.

"It was either a high tolerance of pain or just stupidity," he said. "Maybe both. I was just never the type to lean on someone about my troubles."

"I remember going to a swimming pool at about 13," he recollected. "I was chasing a soccer ball and caught my foot on a wire-mesh basket. I looked down and saw blood on the floor. I thought, I'll dive into the pool and the water will wash it off. Well, I dove in and my big toe started flapping. I took a look and saw that I had a big gash. My toe was almost hanging off. So I went to the first-aid unit, and the guy said, 'Better get this stitched up.' He called an ambulance and I went to the local hospital. The doctor put in about a dozen stitches. Later, I went home with my toe in a big, fat bandage, and the next day I took care of my paper route, same as always. My Mom said, 'How are you?' I said, 'Fine.'"

He had almost lost his toe, and his mother never knew.

So it would go, he decided, in his confrontation with cancer: Nobody is going to take care of this for me, he thought. I'll have to go out and do it for myself.

❦ ❦ ❦

The protocol for chemo was difficult. It called for Griffiths to undergo four cycles of treatments, with three days on as the drugs seeped into his system, and three weeks off to recover from the toxic effects. This would go on again and again, for a total of about three months. But Clive began to form his own agenda. Let's see, he thought as soon as he got wind of this schedule. If I start therapy now, that takes me through April, May, June, and July. He began calculating the immediate consequences for his career with the Comets—and the possibilities of a comeback. Training camp in August and September. Exhibition season in October. Regular season in November.

Meanwhile, the Kansas City Comets embarked on a playoff drive with a long road trip to Phoenix, San Diego, and Los Angeles. Clive wrote his teammates an open letter. "I told the other players that I had a job to do, to fight my cancer, and that they had a job to do, too, to win games and make the playoffs." Coach McBride read the letter to the team before the Phoenix game. He then posted the message on the locker-room bulletin board for all to read.

Clive began chemo on April 14, the first day the Comets competed in the playoffs.

The first drug to enter his bloodstream was cisplatin, a potent, relatively new drug for testicular cancer. It was given in the maximum dosage, along with vinblastine and bleomycin. A few hours later, while Clive and Marylee played Scrabble in his hospital room, his eyes suddenly turned glassy. He broke into a drenching sweat. He began to throw up and kept vomiting almost every 15 minutes. Marylee—now 29 pounds pregnant, ready to give birth any day—gagged from the stench. "He was just retching, holding his belly, curling himself in a ball like a fetus," she said. "All I could do was wipe his forehead and take the bedpans to the bathroom to rinse. I just felt so helpless." Once in the bathroom, she would cry. It was the only place she would let the tears flow. She never cried in front of her husband.

Six days later, Marylee went into labor and entered the hospital. Clive was still weak from his first chemo session; the vomiting had blanched his already pale Welsh complexion to a ghoulish white. He called to ask his friend Mark West to drive him to see Marylee in the hospital. "I wanted to see my baby born," Clive said. "I knew the moment was now and would never happen again." West escorted Clive to the delivery room to witness the birth. And there, at 3:00 a.m., Marylee gave birth to an eight-pound, two-ounce girl, blond and blue-eyed, Meredith Lee.

Clive had so exerted himself in rushing to the hospital and beholding this singular event that the physicians had to usher him, exhausted, to a nearby office and let him lie down on a sofa.

For the next few days, the hospital gave the Griffiths a private room with two single beds so Clive could stay overnight. The nurses would periodically wheel in Meredith so her parents could ogle and coo at the newborn.

❦ ❦ ❦

Clive was still far from finished with the chemo, and he returned three weeks later to the University of Kansas Medical Center for the second of his four treatment sessions. Gradually, as the second chemo dose took hold, the signature curly locks Clive had worn so proudly fell from his scalp in clumps, especially while he showered. Clive finally went to his hairdresser and, all traces of vanity gone, told him to shave him bald.

He continued to grapple with nausea and vomited, violently, day and night. "I just lay there knowing that in a few hours, the vomiting would start," Clive said. "After a while, you would try to throw up and nothing would come out." After a chemo session, it would take him at least three days to regain even a faint appetite. Over one stretch, he went 10 days without consuming any solid food. He forced himself to eat, if only to maintain his stamina and strength, and Marylee prepared protein feasts—milk shakes and anything fattening—for him. Still, the pounds inexorably peeled away from his frame.

Clive lay in bed, listless and constipated. He frequently felt lightheaded and his thoughts rambled. Playing Scrabble, he began to spell nonsense words. His jaw puffed out and ached with pain. His lips and throat blistered, growing so sore and tender that he had to drink liquids through a straw. "All I could do was try to hold on," he said.

After each cycle of chemo, the hospital monitored his blood count, making sure he had enough white cell platelets to stave off infection. Still, the back-to-back operations, combined with the drug therapy, conspired to weaken his condition and leave him susceptible to bacteria. Between chemo sessions, he had to recuperate and conserve his strength for the next round.

When Clive went to the hospital with Marylee for round three, he stopped at the front door, ready to tell Dr. Stevens that he was quitting the chemo. He hated to go to the hospital because the chemo seemed to go on forever, on and on, hour after hour, day after day. He felt vulnerable, and, for the first time, entertained doubts about getting back to the Comets. He asked himself, *God, when is this going to stop?*

In front of the hospital, Clive turned to Marylee and said, "I can't do this again. I really can't."

"Clive, don't be silly, we're halfway there," Marylee answered. "We'll get through it. You've got to."

And on the thrust of this rallying exhortation, Clive forged ahead.

In the three-week intervals between chemo doses, Clive stayed at home with his wife and daughter. "I wanted to look after myself as much as I could," he recalled, "to prevent my illness from being a burden on Marylee. Still, she never let me get away with any special favors. She wanted our lives to take their normal courses and refused to let me feel sorry for myself. She encouraged me to participate in raising the baby as much as possible, because I was right there, recovering at home. She would never say, 'Clive, you look sick as a dog, go lie down on the couch.' Instead, she would say, 'Clive, get yourself up here and feed the baby.'"

Clive lay in bed many a night, fitful and sleepless, anxiety and dread prying open his eyes. His thoughts would race through scenarios of disease and decay. Then he would hear Meredith, from her crib in the nursery, crying for her bottle of warm milk. Marylee would mumble and roll over to climb out of bed for the feeding. More often than not Clive would say, "No, it's okay. I'm awake anyway. Let me go."

It became a point of honor with Clive to perform his parental duties, including changing the occasional diaper, even in the thick of chemo. He found the presence of Meredith to have an effect that was almost medicinal. She buoyed him along through his illness, an extra incentive to get better, a bonus of a reason to live.

In the dead of any given night those first few weeks after her birth, Clive would lean back in the rocking chair in the living room and cradle Meredith in his arms. He would stroke her strawberry-blond hair and peer into her blue eyes. With the bottle of warm milk nuzzled between her lips, he would bend his head over to within inches of her ear. "I want you to know me, Meredith," he would whisper. "I promise you I'm going to live to see you grow up."

After the baby dozed off, Clive could have lowered her back into the crib. Instead, he would keep her safe in his arms and stretch himself out on the sofa. Meredith would clutch his shoulders with her tiny fingers, her cheek soft against his stubbled jaw. Her breath would slow as the milk tranquilized her, and Clive, also calmed, would finally sink into a long, restful night of sleep. In the morning, Marylee would come downstairs and find her husband asleep, nine-pound Meredith, almost marsupial, still atop his once-brawny chest.

❦ ❦ ❦

From the first surgery on, Coach McBride had visited Clive every week, either at his home or in the hospital. Teammate Mark Frederickson would also visit, bringing along his wife, Kathy, often staying for dinner. But since the chemo had begun, the other Comets had stayed away from Clive. The Griffiths had felt outcast, stigmatized.

"It was a shock for the players to see someone so physically fit diagnosed with cancer," Marylee said. "They just had a tough time dealing with it. Not everyone could handle coming to Clive and seeing him lying there all bald and thin. I understand that."

As Griffiths progressed through his chemo regimen, he trained his sights on an ideal vision of himself. The image would start off fuzzy. Then slowly, with the fine-tuning of lucid reverie, he would bring the image into focus. He would see himself reclaiming his spot as a fixture in the starting lineup of the Kansas City Comets.

Dr. Stevens encouraged this quest. He never promised Clive a full recovery, but he told him that, medically, nothing should stop him from bouncing back to play soccer again. The physician let Clive know that, simply put, it was all up to him now. "Clive," Stevens said, "no matter how bad you feel now—as bad as your blood is, as devastated as your body feels—you can be on that field for exhibition season in October."

❦ ❦ ❦

The chemo ended in mid-June. Clives's weight had plummeted from 182 pounds to 157. And soon, he encountered a new setback. In his zeal to rehabilitate himself, he tried nine holes of golf—without a green light from Drs. Kurtz or Stevens. No problem, he thought. It's just golf. But when he got home from the links, he realized that he was sniffling and his nose was dripping nonstop. The next day, Stevens discovered that Clive had a perilously low white-blood-cell count, almost zero, and ran a high risk of mortal infection. Clive had to be quarantined for a few days, until his white-cell count returned to normal. Marylee had to wear a mask when she visited Clive in the hospital.

The quarantine served as a grave warning, at least for the short term: no exertion whatsoever. Not even a half round of golf.

After a while, though, Clive began training for the 1983–84 soccer season. At first, he jogged slowly and briefly around town.

He would run a quarter-mile, rest a minute, and maybe log another quarter-mile. He gradually intensified his exercise program, each week running harder and farther, testing the limits of his endurance. He ran once a week, then twice, and finally three times. Soon he was going a mile, then a mile-and-a-half, and even adding a sprint at the end of a workout session. But after a few weeks, he still weighed 15 pounds less than usual and lacked his characteristic muscularity.

Clive was one of 10 defenders vying for eight spots on the Comets' roster, and nothing was guaranteed for anyone. It was a question of whether Clive would start games or warm the bench and fill in for others.

"I decided that, no matter what, I was going to be in training camp," Clive recalled. "I had another battle to fight besides cancer—staying on the team. I had played soccer professionally almost half my life. It was my livelihood. It was all I knew."

During the summer, Clive worked out on his own. "Clive had been a handsome, well-built man with long, flowing hair," Charlie Carey, a neighbor and teammate, said. "But now he had no hair and he looked like a refugee from a prison camp. It definitely took courage and humility for him to come out in public looking like that." By the end of August, Clive was participating in scrimmages with the Comets. Such practice sessions were much more strenuous than training solo because he was pushed around so much.

In September, a short-haired, pared-down Clive Griffiths made it to training camp. Full of himself again, he occasionally goofed around on the playing field. At one point he bobbed around in front of teammate Gino Schiraldi like a prizefighter—mockingly, with fists raised, but smiling—as if to demonstrate his readiness for the battle that still lay ahead. But Clive made a point, in wind sprints and longer runs, of keeping up with the other players. "I always felt pressure to appear to be 100 percent," he said. Slowly, his legs again turned sturdy and supple, and he regained his wind, his rhythm, and his confidence. His hair grew back to its previous state of lushness. "It's like Sampson in the Bible," Clive said. "As his hair grew longer, he got stronger." In practice games, Clive ran and kicked well, attacking on defense. He heard a familiar refrain resonate in his head. *Win the ball.* It was like a siren song. *Win the ball.*

But sometimes he seemed tentative, out of character for his slash-and-burn style. He refrained from carrying out certain tactical defensive specialties, most notably his trademark slide tackle.

Clive continued to volunteer for charitable organizations. To Marylee, it seemed that at every turn, someone, usually a friend or relative of a cancer patient, would call with a request. Would Clive talk to a patient, visit a hospital, give a speech? "If you asked him to do 100 appearances in the community, he'd say, 'Sure,'" Marylee said. "He never said no to anyone, and I felt that sometimes he should."

With training camp about a month under way, however, his spiritual largesse got the best of Clive. He went to Topeka to give a speech at an American Cancer Society banquet, but it was evidently one speech too many. While standing at the podium, he broke into a heavy, feverish sweat. Pneumonia, it turned out. He spent the next three days taking antibiotics at the University of Kansas City Medical Center.

"I would tell myself, Let's just wait and see," Clive recalled. "And then something bad would happen, and I would go on, and something else bad would happen." God, he thought. I wonder if I'll make it in time. I'd better. If I miss this season, my career is over. "But I knew I would survive. If I could get through chemotherapy, I would get through pneumonia."

True to form, Clive came out on the field on October 3 for the first Comets exhibition game of the season. But McBride felt no small concern about the well-being of his returning captain. McBride was so worried about Clive's cell count, so nervous about pushing him hard enough to force a relapse of pneumonia, that he babied him a bit, limiting his participation in practice sessions. "Okay," he would bark at the team, "everyone take two laps." Then he would turn to Clive and say, "Clive, you take it easy. Take your time."

Clive, wanting no pity or special privileges, called to consult with Dr. Stevens.

"Ron," Clive said over the phone, "my coach is treating me as if I'm still a cancer patient. He's worried I'll have problems doing what I could do before. He's holding me back because he's afraid the workouts are going to harm me."

"I'll call him," Stevens said.

Quickly obliging his patient, Stevens called McBride and told him that he should let Clive exert himself to the extent he wished to. He reassured the coach that the training would inflict no harm on him and that Clive would surely have the sense to stop if he felt the need. Under no circumstances, the physician said, should McBride feel duty-bound to treat the athlete as if he were still afflicted with a disease. Under no circumstances, Stevens added, should the coach hold it against Clive that he had had pneumonia—or, for that matter, cancer.

For Clive, this bid to come back was not only a personal issue but also a general crusade on behalf of cancer patients. If the Comets ever hinted that he had to leave because of his cancer, he believed, it would be a symbolic slap in the face to all cancer patients.

"Cancer patients face discrimination in looking for a job," Clive said. "A personnel executive at a corporation might say, 'Oh, we see you had cancer.' They're afraid you might get sick again and send their insurance premiums soaring. Or one day you might roll over at your desk and die. My knowledge of that kind of prejudice in the marketplace was definitely a factor that motivated me to come back. I wanted to make sure that, no matter what, I would not get cut or traded because I was a cancer patient."

❦ ❦ ❦

The Comets opened the season on November 4 in Kemper Arena, against the Wichita Wings. As the announcer introduced the home team, the players cantered onto the field, accompanied by flashing lights and bursts of billowing theatrical smoke. Then out trotted Clive, hands raised triumphantly over his head. A spotlight beamed down and he hugged his teammates, and the fans whooped and hooted his name. "Clive! Clive! Clive!"

Alas, he watched the contest from the bench as the Comets clipped the Wings, 5–4.

About two weeks later, the Comets faced Phoenix, and Clive started his first regular-season game in eight months. The Comets heralded his entrance onto the field with an announcement over the public-address system, his name echoing out into the stands. The 14,000 fans in attendance stood in tribute, roaring a long, throaty cheer for the team captain. Clive, ever reluctant to revel in the role of hero, signaled his appreciation with a simple wave. I'm not here to take bows, he thought. I'm not here to do a song and dance. I'm here to play soccer.

As usually happens in soccer, a sport with few built-in breaks in action, Clive shuttled on and off the field. But he got his minutes. Three minutes in, three minutes out, then back in again. In the first half, he blocked three shots and even tried a shot on goal, rousing the fans to cheers with each effort. Then, in pursuit of a Phoenix dribbler, he barreled into his patented slide tackle, retrieving the ball for the Comets in one fell swoop, and the Kemper Arena crowd stood for Number 5 again, hailing him with approval and admiration. "That slide tackle was a statement," Marylee said. "He wanted to prove to the team that he was still the same player as before. And he made his point."

Clive played only briefly in the next game, but two days later, against the Pittsburgh Spirit, he played again, demonstrating exemplary defense. With the Comets trailing, 3–0, he led the team back to a tie and sent the contest into overtime. Then, in the sudden-death period, he fed Mark Frederickson the assist that won the game.

As the season progressed, Clive stayed in games for longer and longer stretches. A month into the season, Comets president Tracey Leiweke felt moved to say, "I get a little chill every time I see Clive on the field. A lot of us feared we'd never see him in a uniform again. But we must have underestimated his spirit."

One night, with the team on the road riding a 12-game winning streak, coach McBride approached Clive in a hotel restaurant for a private talk. "Clive," he said, "I'm glad you got your doctor to call me back in exhibition season. I was paranoid about your cancer, and I owe you an apology."

"Why?" Clive asked.

"Because I made it tough on you. I want to apologize for all the doubts I had about you and for all the problems I put you through. I had my doubts you would come back. But you've done it. I want to reassure you that you've done a great job. I just hope you'll forgive me."

And forgive him Clive did.

All season long, Clive felt good and clean and strong. By March 1984—a year after the diagnosis of his cancer—he had competed in 32 games and blocked 46 shots, with six assists. The Comets had compiled an 18–14 record. By the end of the 1983–84 season, he had played in 46 of 48 games for the club, racking up 67 blocks, eight assists and one goal. In April the Comets clinched a playoff berth and challenged St. Louis for a division title.

Ever since the initial diagnosis, Clive had set goals. Get through the orchiectomy and the lymphadenectomy. See Meredith born healthy. Make it through the quarantine and the pneumonia. Get into shape. Reach training camp. Start the exhibition season. Make the lineup for the regular season. Finish the season. Get into the playoffs. And Clive had met every demand.

❦ ❦ ❦

In 1985, Clive Griffiths retired as a soccer player. His athletic career had ended, more or less, as he had wished it might—on his own terms. "I never stopped playing because I was sick," he said. "I went out on top, playing very well. And I should thank God that fighting to stay on the team made me stronger against cancer."

Comets owner David Shoenstadt signed Clive to a three-year, personal services contract. Soon, Clive applied the same work ethic that had succeeded for him on the playing field to his job in the front office. He stayed late and never missed a day, never even took a vacation. The Iron Man, even in jacket and tie. For Griffiths, who had left school at 15, this job was the equivalent of a college education, with a major in management.

While an executive with the team, Clive called the Kansas City chapter of the American Cancer Society, the national voluntary health agency fighting cancer through research, education, and service for cancer patients and families. As an honorary board member, he already had attended many banquets, auctions, presentations, and fund-raisers for the local ACS branch. Now he met its director for lunch to ask to do more.

"Those functions I went to are important, of course," Clive said. "You go to a ceremony. You're a face, a public figure. You smile, you shake hands. You go through the routine. People say, 'Oh look, here's the soccer player who had cancer.' But what sort of impact was I really making? Anybody can smile and shake hands. I needed to be more effective. After awhile, the director and I realized that my role lay in education. I like to teach. Over the years I'd developed a rapport with kids, at soccer clinics and seminars. I'd always loved going to the hospital to give the sick kids a smile. I believe it's important for people to know about testicular cancer, to overcome all the ignorance, and I needed a chance to tell my story."

On behalf of the American Cancer Society, Clive began to speak about the disease at high schools across Kansas. Eventually, he helped assemble an educational videotape about cancer prevention and testicular self-examination to present to the high schools at which he spoke.

"I always said to myself, even during the chemo, that some day I would probably have the opportunity to give back something positive," Clive said. "And that's what keeps me motivated to exercise my power of communication. I've probably gotten more out of implementing this program than I ever got out of playing soccer. Kids love the program, and a lot of good has come out of it. Boys have gone home to Mom and said, 'We heard this great talk today about cancer.' Or they say, 'Mom, I think I've got a problem here,' and they get it checked out."

Until Clive came along, few survivors of testicular cancer wanted to acknowledge, in public, what they had gone through. Most recovering patients suffered shame and embarrassment and a sense of maligned masculinity. As with breast cancer years earlier, cancer of the testes was enshrouded in a cult of silence. But in talking to teenage boys, Clive helped bring the disease out of the closet.

Nancy Moylan, Director of Public Education, District Four, in the Missouri Division of the American Cancer Society, has worked with Clive on his educational programs over the years. "He reached out to the community and spread the word," she said. "He has a bulldog passion for getting the job done. He makes people believe they can move mountains, and the American Cancer Society is forever grateful to him."

Said Clive, "Ten years from now, a kid will remember that some athlete came along and talked about testicular cancer, and he'll remember to check himself out," Clive continued. "Or the person I talked to in high school may have a chance to help a friend of his. Somebody, somewhere, will be exposed to what I said. We all have in our hands the power to communicate. I hope that my listeners pass on my knowledge and cause a boy to catch the disease early—early enough to save him the trouble of radical surgery and chemotherapy. Early enough, maybe, to help save a life."

Clive became a national spokesperson for the American Cancer Society. For his educational efforts, he was invited to the White House in May 1988 as one of 57 distinguished cancer survivors. There, at a ceremony in the Oval Office, he received the highest honor the society bestows, which is its Courage Award, from President George Bush.

❦ ❦ ❦

Clive remained in the Comets front office for four years. After he left the club in 1989, he went into business for himself, starting on a shoestring investment of $100. His venture, International Soccer Camps, is a summer-camp instructional program for children aged six to 18. By 1990, Clive had set up 46 soccer camps in nine states, as far east as Pennsylvania and Virginia, as far south as Florida and Texas. He had recruited coaches from England, Wales, Ireland, France, and Brazil to manage the camps, which featured specialized outposts specifically for scorers, goalkeepers, and defenders. It's a one-man operation, built through elbow grease, salesmanship, and organizational talents.

Clive also formed the Sports Travel Network, which takes U.S. children aged 10 to 18 to tour several European countries and compete in soccer. By the summer of 1990, he had recruited 4,000 children. He usually takes teams to play in Germany, England, Scotland, Wales, and the Netherlands. Through these tours, the kids get some otherwise unobtainable international seasoning. "The game is tougher over there, and Europeans have more experience," Griffiths said. "The United States is still young and raw when it comes to soccer. This tour gives American youngsters an opportunity to compete on an international stage—and to experience the culture of Europe."

He continues as president of both operations. Today, the Griffiths' family room is decorated, not only with soccer memorabilia and awards and trophies Clive has won over the years, but also—most prized of all—trophies bestowed on the teams of youngsters he has coached and taken to Europe.

ೇ ೇ ೇ

Every week during his last training camp and exhibition season, Clive diligently returned to the University of Kansas Medical Center to see Dr. Ron Stevens for chest X-rays and blood-cell counts. After the Comets made the league playoffs, Clive continued to see Dr. Stevens monthly. The follow-up visits became bimonthly after a year, quarterly after two, biannually after three, then annually.

The fifth-year checkup is considered a milestone for cancer patients, an emblem of cure or remission, and Clive reached this watershed with relief and gratitude. After his fifth-year checkup, he had the option of bypassing further visits. Still, just to be certain, he went in for a sixth-year exam.

Every year, Casey Regan sends the Griffiths a Christmas card. Once in a while, she sends Clive a fan letter thanking him again for his visits to her and wishing him good health. One year she bought a holiday ornament as a present for Meredith Griffiths. In 1990, Casey, like Clive, received an Ambassador of Hope Award from the American Cancer Society. Then a fully grown 18-year-old, the baby fat and the braces and the pimples long since faded into memory, she was handed the award, fittingly, by none other than Clive himself.

"My survival is no mystery to me," Clive reflected. "I discovered the pain in my testicle in the early stages, before the tumor could creep into my lungs and chest. I was very fortunate to have detected it early. I also received a very potent, very effective, chemo drug called cisplatin. Until about 1975, physicians had no drug—no cisplatin—for treatment of testicular cancer. Back then, testicular cancer often killed people in six months. The disease might have killed me, too. But thanks to research funded with dollars donated by the public, we have developed drugs like cisplatin to combat the disease. And people like me have gotten a second chance.

"I think athletes have an advantage against cancer. And not only because they're in better physical condition. Sure, they're conscientious about taking care of themselves physically. Being in good physical condition definitely helped me recover—my doctors told me that. But there's no doubt you also have to be in good mental condition. You have to keep your mind right. An athlete has the powerful concentration and willpower to deal with pain and fatigue. You learn discipline, and that can see you through cancer as well. For me, keeping a positive attitude was the most important aspect of beating cancer. I'll say this: Not everyone can be an athlete, but everyone can develop the right mental condition.

"I heard a sermon once where the preacher said that God puts giants in your path for you to overcome in order to grow. It's true. I've seen those Goliaths all my life. Getting past those obstacles has very much deepened my faith in God. Where else are you going to turn for help? Of course, you have to listen to your doctors and have faith in what they tell you and do what you have to do to get through your treatments. But you realize a doctor can do only so much. You also turn to God and ask Him what you should do. Maybe, after all, my cancer was a sign from God. He just said, 'Hey, you're going to suffer for a while, but in the end, your purpose is to do a real job for somebody.' I feel I've survived to help educate people about beating cancer, to put out the word that 50 percent of all cancers are curable. If people are encouraged and inspired by my situation, then it was all worth it."

❦ ❦ ❦

Clive became close to Meredith after leaving the Comets, working as he does out of an office at home. If his daughter stayed home from school sick, he brought her muffins and tea. They played Monopoly and talked. But he also cultivated in the bashful Meredith a spirit of independence that harked back, if dimly, to his days in Pontypridd. On certain days, he let her answer his business phone. She joined a baseball league, and in third grade, even entered a talent show, taking on the role of ringleader in making the necessary costumes. Her teacher at school noticed that, somewhere along the line, Meredith had changed. She was talking more, coming out of her shell. Through her father, she had gained a stronger sense of importance.

Clive also took her to speeches he gave for the American

Cancer Society. He explained that the society raised money for research in preventing and treating cancer. He could never forget—nor will he ever—that his daughter was born while he fought to live.

One day Meredith, then about 7 years old, asked Marylee, "Did Daddy ever have cancer?"

Her mother said, "Yes."

"Where?"

"You've seen his scar, right?" His second surgery had left him with a scar from his breastbone to his groin.

And that was that as far as her curiosity went—until about six months later. Meredith had begun to wonder why she had no brothers or sisters, and tried to piece together the puzzle. As the family of three sat at the kitchen table, Marylee delicately explained that Clive could no longer produce sperm and that without sperm you cannot create a child.

"What about me?" Meredith asked. "How did I get here?"

"Well, Meredith," Clive answered, "you came along just in the nick of time."

Chapter 4

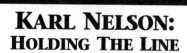

KARL NELSON:
HOLDING THE LINE

If you ask Karl Nelson about his role in Super Bowl XXI, he'll give you a short answer. After all, he scored no touchdowns, kicked no field goals, and intercepted no passes in the Rose Bowl in Pasadena, California, on January 25, 1987. Neither Wheaties nor Disneyland approached him for commercial endorsements after the contest between the New York Giants and the Denver Broncos. If you ask Nelson that question, he might even shrug. "My role for the Giants in the 1987 Super Bowl?" the mustachioed Nelson would answer in his sepulchral basso profundo. "Why, I played right tackle."

How true. The 285-pound, 27-year-old played right tackle, as always, right on the offensive line. And, as ever, he had a hand in almost every point the Giants scored. With his blocking, quarterback Phil Simms hit a six-yard pass for a touchdown in the first quarter. With Number 63 slamming defenders, tight end Mark Bavaro broke loose to catch a 13-yard pass in the end zone. As Nelson pried open cracks in the Denver defensive line, halfback Joe Morris rammed ahead for two quick, short-yardage touchdowns.

And when the game ended, the Giants had whipped Denver, 39–20, the team claiming its first National Football League (NFL) championship in 30 years. Karl Nelson played right tackle for New York in Super Bowl XXI, all right, and now he and the Giants had captured the world championship. The right tackle had tasted the ultimate triumph in the game of football.

❦ ❦ ❦

Seven months later, sweet turned to sour. In August 1987, the New York Giants gathered in New Jersey for summer training camp. Nelson came in as strong as ever, thanks to a rigorous off-season workout program. But when he blocked on the line, he felt a sharp pain in his left shoulder. Every time he thrust both arms out in front of him, his left shoulder seemed to slide in and out of its socket. Without this double stiff-arm to impede onrushing defenders, he could block forcefully only with his right arm. Being right tackle, he found himself hard-pressed to protect the inside of the offensive line and especially vulnerable to the pass rush.

Nelson complained about his shoulder pain to Dr. Russell Warren, the Giants' long-time team physician, after an exhibition game against the New England Patriots. Warren found an uncommon dislocation: the head of Nelson's left humerus bone had popped out of the back of his shoulder joint, causing inflammation. The orthopedist recommended arthroscopic surgery. Nelson believed that if that was what he had to do to get ready for the season, then that was what he would do, and quickly. How often does one get the opportunity to defend a Super Bowl title? Warren scheduled what is known as a "scope," to remove bone spurs in the shoulder, at the Hospital for Special Surgery in Manhattan.

On Tuesday, August 18, in preparing for surgery, Nelson received an obligatory chest X-ray. Dr. Warren found the results troubling. "We found something on your X-ray," he told Nelson the next day. He showed his patient the film, pointing out an unidentified dark blur in the chest. "I see a real problem. Something funny has shown up."

"What are you talking about?" Nelson asked Warren. "Let's just get this scope done."

"No," Warren said. "I see something suspicious. We have to take another look at this. I want to run some tests and do a biopsy."

I'm a football player, Nelson thought. Nothing is going to be wrong with me. He considered himself indestructible. As a football player, you had to. And if you were a hulking ramrod of an offensive lineman, programmed to function as a human battering ram, you had all the more reason to. The job called for the kind of mindset dictating that nothing gets through you.

Still, Nelson underwent additional chest X-rays and a CAT scan the next day. After Warren examined the films, he consulted with other physicians and talked to Nelson. He had found a fist-sized mass, six inches in diameter, in the lymph nodes to the right of his breastplate. "Tomorrow, we have to do some exploratory surgery," he told the lineman. "The operation is called a thoracotomy. We just want to take out the mass and see what's going on in there."

Nelson had no idea why this was happening, and neither did

his wife, Heidi, home with their 2-year-old daughter, Brittany. He had gone in for arthroscopic surgery on his left shoulder, and now the doctors were going to carve open his chest and pluck out a foreign object of undetermined origin. Warren told Heidi that she would be better off waiting at home during the surgery.

On Thursday, orderlies wheeled Karl through an underground corridor at New York Hospital to the operating room. It was a major undertaking to gain access to the mass in Nelson's chest. Thoracic surgeon Dr. Arthur Okinaka made an 18-inch incision under Nelson's right arm that stretched back across the top of his shoulder blade. Okinaka let his right lung collapse and removed a five-inch section of his bottom right rib. Then the surgeon sliced away at the mass with painstaking care and took out a section of it. He dispatched the biopsy to the pathology lab for a report.

It turned out to be malignant.

Dr. Warren phoned Heidi. "It's cancer," he said.

Heidi cried hysterically, frightened that Karl would soon die. She rushed to see her husband, assuming that Warren had already relayed the news to him. "I was scared," she recalled. "Scared about losing a husband, scared for myself, scared about my child losing a father. I freaked out a little."

Heidi reached Karl only a few hours after he emerged from the recovery room. As she leaned over his bed, he lay groggy from anesthesia, a tube coming out of his chest to clear his lungs of excess fluid.

The next day, Dr. David Wolf, an oncologist at New York Hospital, gave the football player the official diagnosis: he had Hodgkin's disease, a form of lymphatic cancer. Wolf reassured him that Hodgkin's is the most treatable of all lymphomas and, if detected early, has a 90 percent cure rate.

Ninety percent, Nelson thought. He liked the sound of that percentage. The numbers are on my side. He mulled over the figure for a few seconds. I'm probably not going to die. He took a deep breath, relieved to hear of his high prospects for survival. All right. I can live with that, he thought. He again breathed deeply and turned to Wolf.

"Okay," Nelson said. "That's good news. Now, what do I have to do to get better?"

"You'll need some treatment," Wolf said.

"Can I get back to playing football?"

"No," the physician said. "Probably not."

Oh yes I can, Nelson thought. He was right tackle for the Super Bowl champion New York Giants, and he had a job to do.

❦ ❦ ❦

Karl Nelson grew up playing sports in DeKalb, Illinois. He just followed the seasons. In the fall, he played on the football team, stationed on the offensive line; in winter, basketball, as a center; in spring, baseball, as a catcher. That's how it went for him in DeKalb all through junior high and high school.

He lettered in three sports, but he never saw himself as an athlete per se; he was a student who happened to play sports. Nelson gravitated toward academic pursuits rather than focus single-mindedly on sports. He organized a schedule to see him through the dual demands of the classroom and the ballfield. Classes all day. Athletic practice after school, whether football, basketball, or baseball. Homework every night. And he stuck to it.

Nelson recognized early on that he was neither a brilliant student nor a particularly gifted athlete. Nothing would come easy for him, nobody was going to hand him the holy grail. So he became the kind of kid who worked hard at everything. He cultivated a sense of responsibility rare for a teenager and, along with it, a habit of planning everything down to the last detail. He believed that discipline, preparation and sacrifice would bring him success. The result was that in every class throughout high school except two, he scored an "A."

But if anatomy is destiny, then Nelson seemed fated to establish his identity less as a student than as an athlete. In the eighth grade, at the age of 14, he already stood 5 feet, 8 inches, taller than all his classmates, and seemed a natural to take advantage of his superior size, no matter what the game. He sprouted four inches a year, reaching six feet tall as a high school freshman, 6 feet, 4 inches as a sophomore and, as a junior, attaining his full, final height of a shade over 6 feet, 6 inches. He stood head and shoulders above everyone else in school, a lanky 200-pounder with a narrow torso, wide hips and thick legs.

In baseball, Nelson switched from catcher to first base because the umpire behind home plate had trouble seeing over him. He started varsity basketball, imagining that someday he might play the game for a medium-sized college. In football he tried tight end and defensive end before finding a home in his senior year on the offensive line at tackle, now weighing in at a much more substantial 220 pounds. Coaches from the universities of Notre Dame and Nebraska and Michigan began to scramble for his services, offering him football scholarships.

Nelson elected to attend Iowa State University. There, given his aptitude toward the analytical, he majored in industrial engineering. He took school so seriously that only once during football season did he go out with friends on a weeknight, and then it was to split a pitcher of beer with two friends in his senior year.

To him, football was not only a physical enterprise but also an engineering proposition, a set of equations and theorems to be cranked out. He devoured the playbook, where diagrams spelled out everything in black and white. He could quickly grasp the relationship among components, identify the variables, calculate the permutations. He laid everything out, step by step, in his mind. If this happens, then that happens. Cause and effect, action and reaction, like a set of dominoes poised to tip over at the flick of a finger. Nelson believed that if you went along systematically, from Step A to Step B, you would get where you wanted to go.

It turned out to be true. Nelson earned honors as an Academic all-American at Iowa State. He also was voted to the Big Eight conference All-Decade Team of the 1980s.

He never intended to play professional football until his coach, Donnie Duncan, took him aside in the spring of his senior year and told him he could. Nelson had doubts about going pro. He told Duncan he planned to earn his keep as an engineer. He figured it like this: he had always gotten accolades by exploiting his body, and now he wanted to let his brain do more of the talking. Then Duncan told Nelson how much money he could earn in the National Football League. Nelson paused for a moment. Well, he thought, maybe I'll use my body a little longer.

In the 1983 NFL draft, the New York Giants picked Nelson in the third round (sweetening the deal with a $90,000 signing bonus). The young engineering student was going to compete with the big boys.

❦ ❦ ❦

Hodgkin's disease is a common form of lymphoma, a malignancy of the lymph system. Named for 19th-century English physician Thomas Hodgkin, who discovered it, the disease annually affects about 9,000 people in the United States. Most patients are 20 to 35 years of age, or, less likely, over 50. The most common early sign of the disease is a painless swelling of the lymph glands, most often those on either side of the neck, but sometimes in the armpit or groin. Other possible symptoms include persistent fatigue, recurrent high fever, sweating at night, severe itching; pain in the back, legs or abdomen; nausea or vomiting, loss of weight, and bone pain. The disease may also appear, as in the case of Karl Nelson, with no symptoms at all.

Its cause remains unknown.

The disease first manifests itself in the lymph system, the network of tiny vessels lining the blood vessels that manufacture infection-fighting antibodies and connect the bean-sized glands known as lymph nodes. In Hodgkin's, these nodes generally become progressively larger. At the same time, white blood cells, mostly lymphocytes—critical as a defense against poison, bacteria, and other infections—grow abnormally. The aberrant cells multiply so much that they crowd out and impair the function of the normal white cells. Patients become susceptible to infections and anemia and, in advanced cases, to tumors in the lymph nodes themselves.

The size and severity of a growth are most accurately pinpointed by biopsy, the surgical removal of a thin slice of a suspicious node, so a pathologist can examine it under a microscope for the presence of malignant cells. If malignancy is confirmed, the doctor calls for additional diagnostic procedures, such as blood tests, CAT scans, X-rays of the lymph system, radioactive scanning of the bone and bone marrow, and tests of kidney and liver function.

Hodgkin's in its early stages is typically treated with super-voltage radiation targeted at shrinking the enlarged lymph nodes. Such radiotherapy may also be directed to all lymph nodes in adjacent regions of the torso. Side effects can include cotton-mouth, sore throat, fatigue, and a drop in the number of red blood cells and platelets, the fragments in the blood that help prevent bleeding.

Treatment for the disease may involve chemotherapy, either alone or in combination with radiotherapy. Sometimes radiation comes first, then, if the disease returns, doctors turn to chemo. But the disease grows slowly and takes a long time to spread to vital organs such as the lungs, liver, spleen, intestines, spinal cord, or brain. In the event the disease is already advanced, the therapy of choice is often chemo involving two different four-drug combinations, the most common being nitrogen mustard, vincristine, procarbazine, and prednisone. This combination results in complete remission in 80 percent of cases.

About one in six Americans who develop Hodgkin's— approximately 1,500 patients a year—die from it. If untreated, the disease is usually fatal. The major long-term risk of radiation and chemotherapy is impaired reproductive ability (permanent sterility for males and females). The good news is that survival rates have improved greatly in recent years. In 1955, the average Hodgkin's patient died within 30 months of onset. Today, more than 90 percent of cases detected early can be arrested, and about 50 percent of those diagnosed and treated in the later stages of the disease go on to live productively. If the condition is confined to a single lymph node, the chance of survival is highest; the odds decline if the disease spreads.

The question in Karl Nelson's case was, had the doctors caught the disease early enough to assure his longevity?

❦ ❦ ❦

Blocking—that's how Karl Nelson made his living for the New York Giants. He blocked. If the team called for a pass, Nelson fended off opponents rushing the quarterback. If the Giants wanted a run, he drove defenders back like a snow plow, opening the line for the running back. Mainly, he pushed and shoved, his job to engage in hand-to-hand combat, all slams and grunts. Dig in. Plow through. Hold the line.

Life on the line in the NFL was not easy. An offensive lineman never got the glory of bolting to daylight on an end sweep or diving for a catch in the end zone or fading back into the pocket to unleash the bomb. No, it was a blue-collar job, pretty much menial labor when you got right down to it. You lived down in the trenches, doing the dirty work, just another grunt. Nelson knew that. Along with his fellow grunts on the Giants—Chris Godfrey, Billy Ard, Bart Oates, and Brad Benson—Nelson realized that few fans watched the line and fewer still understood it. He accepted the reality that once the play began, everyone watched the ball, not the blockers. An offensive lineman heard his name announced in a game only after he committed a holding penalty, never for setting a key block. As Nelson put it, "If you do your job well, others—the quarterback and the running back—succeed."

In his first season as a starter for the Giants, Nelson had a short fuse. He took it personally if a defensive lineman either swung around him on a play or, worse still, slammed the halfback for a loss or sacked the quarterback. He would stomp around after such an event, cursing himself for blowing the coverage.

Finally, Giants coach Bill Parcells took the rookie aside. Better watch that temper, the coach told him. Never let the other guy know he's gotten the better of you. Showing your anger and frustration could give him an incentive to come on harder, go for the kill. No, Parcells advised Nelson, keep quiet after every play, turn around and return to the huddle. Just go about your business. Parcells delivered this message to Nelson whenever he erupted. The player was a quick study. After only a few games, the lesson took. And in 1984, he won a spot on the NFL All-Rookie Team.

Nelson trained in the weight room like a scientist, still the engineering student at heart. Other offensive linemen, with bigger upper bodies than his, more mesomorphic in design, could muscle defenders with their shoulders, chest, and arms. But Nelson could never get away with that. Besides, he knew that, biomechanically, you applied the most effective leverage against defenders not with your torso but with your legs, the lowest possible center of gravity. So while other linemen performed bench presses to build mass in the torso, Nelson concentrated on power cleans—squatting low, his behind just inches off the floor, to hoist as much as 365 pounds to his waist in one swift explosion of energy—to strengthen his lower body, chiefly his lower back, buttocks, thighs, ankles, and feet. He engineered his physique for maximum output. Other Giants bench-pressed 40, 50 pounds more than they power-cleaned; Nelson did just the opposite.

As he had at Iowa State, Nelson relied heavily on technique. In studying game films, he observed how opposing linemen moved and, equally telling, how he reacted. It was real important in the pros to do your homework. In the Big Eight, he might face two or three formidable defensive linemen in a year. But in the NFL, *everyone* was good; any defender could blow past you on any given play in any game, and you had to have your technique down cold. On the offensive line, pure physical prowess brought fewer benefits than technique. You had to control your moves, choreograph almost every step. Nelson picked up a reputation as a thinker. He sat with his fellow offensive linemen for hours and talked about technique. Cause and effect, Step A to step B.

Parcells took exception to this view. He saw that Nelson played to the level of his competition, accomplishing no more than necessary to do the job. If Nelson rammed a defender back a yard or two to spring loose his running back, that was good enough. As much as the coach admired proper technique, he really preferred to see a little unadulterated aggression out there. Again, he counseled Nelson. Stop being so intellectual about it, Parcells told him. Show me some attitude.

"He'd get on me about my being too systematic, too technique-oriented," Nelson said. If he could drive a defender back three or four yards on a play and then pancake him—demoralizing him in the process—so much the better. "Your technique can be perfect, and you can still get your butt run over," Nelson said. "Parcells pushed me to keep my emotions internal, yet get cranked up enough to do the job. He told me I was too much 'if-I-take-this-step-then-this-happens-but-if-I-take-that-step-then-that-happens.' Sometimes you just need a kick in the ass. He would say that at some point you have to get it done—decide the hell with technique and strap it up and go whale on somebody."

Nelson compromised. From then on, he struck a balance between the textbook intricacies of technique and the ugly imperatives of brute ferocity. In short, he copped a major attitude. He visualized a defender beating him to the ball, exploiting this fear to psyche himself, then reversed the scenario and saw himself getting on the guy like a bad rash. He went through this drill and came to relish the competition, the in-your-face, me-against-you stuff.

Every year in the NFL, Nelson improved incrementally. By lifting weights, he added 10 to 15 pounds of muscle to his body each season until he peaked at a weight of 285. By practicing technique, he pushed and shoved with increasing exactitude. And by psyching himself up enough, he got the job done every Sunday. From 1984 to 1986—three full seasons—the Giants started him at tackle in every game, 55 consecutive starts. Once, he sprained an ankle, but Parcells told him, "Karl, you're not allowed to get hurt—we have no backup for you."

All the defensive linemen in the league came to respect him. Strong, smart, and tough—Karl Nelson, with discipline, preparation, and sacrifice, had become the real deal.

❦ ❦ ❦

After the thoracotomy, he went without solid food, just lemon swabs to freshen his mouth, for six days. For three of those days, nurses had to help him out of bed. Then Heidi took him home for a week, only for the doctors to call him back in. He underwent another CAT scan and magnetic resonance imaging. Dr. Wolf had caught the Hodgkin's early, at Stage I, the tumor still localized, Nelson's shot at a full recovery excellent. But nothing was certain. As a precaution, Dr. Wolf ordered another operation: a splenectomy, the removal of his spleen, combined with a laparotomy, the excision of a piece of his liver, kidney and lymph nodes for a biopsy.

"By now, I realized this was not as trivial as I had originally thought," Nelson recalled. "Two major surgeries within two weeks. They were slicing me open and putting tubes in my chest and stapling me shut. I thought, 'Whoa, something is not right here. What's wrong with this picture?'"

Warren told Parcells that Nelson had cancer, and the coach informed the team. A fellow Super Bowl champion had cancer.

"The team was shaken up," Nelson said. "Football players are used to being indestructible, and all of a sudden one of us was diagnosed with cancer. The reality of it slapped everyone in the face."

Teammates, aware of his cancer, whispered among themselves about the disease, out of earshot from Nelson, and gradually withdrew from him. "Teammates never want to associate with someone who is disabled and therefore unproductive," Nelson said. "If you have stopped helping the team, guys will pull away." Still, fellow linemen Chris Godfrey and George Martin and line coach Harry Hoaglin visited him in the hospital.

Two weeks later, Nelson began radiation therapy, to attack any vestiges of disease in his chest. On a Monday morning, he drove his Chevy S-10 from his home in Montvale, New Jersey to the Memorial Sloan-Kettering Cancer Center in Manhattan, a 70-minute trip. He had a 9:45 a.m. appointment with the radiologist.

He lay on his back on a hard table, and technicians tattooed 16 black-dye pinpoints strategically across his chest, underarms, neck, and back, the marks intended to direct radiation to key points on his body. A customized lead shield was placed over his vital organs for protection. Then a device called a high-energy linear accelerator blasted 180 rads at the targeted areas for 35 seconds. Nelson heard a click and a hum, then another click as the machine switched off. He flipped over and received the same treatment on his upper back. The whole procedure took only a minute or two. He felt nothing. But sometimes, as the device emitted its buzz, he imagined he smelled something burning.

Nelson originally expected to follow this regimen for five days a week, Monday through Friday, for four weeks, receiving 20 radiation treatments. But after a month, Dr. Wolf recommended he keep going, to destroy any lingering cancer cells. "Let's make sure we get it all," the player agreed.

Nelson stayed home for a week, to give his blood count a chance to rise back to near normal levels, then went back for more radiation therapy. As expected, he suffered the usual side effects. Damage to his salivary glands erased his sense of taste and created a case of cotton-mouth. He lost hair along the back of his head, a half-moon mark left just above his neck. Worst of all, the radiation tired him out. "It drained the hell out of me," he said.

Nelson went on the Injured Reserve list, plunging headlong into what players call the IR Zone, in which the teammate in extremis suddenly turns persona non grata. "When I got back to the Giants for visits, the team had no idea how to react, so they showed no reaction at all," Nelson recalled. "A lot of guys had no idea how to deal with me, so they just decided not to. If you're even seen standing next to a guy on IR, you're concerned the coach will perceive you as nonproductive."

Veteran linebacker Harry Carson, playing his final season, turned this hokum about the IR Zone into a joke. With Nelson on IR, Carson would say, real loud, right in front of everyone in the locker room, "Hey, Karl! Hey, buddy, how you doing? How you doing today? I'll still talk to you, buddy." Coach Bill Parcells kept tabs on the stricken lineman, sympathetically so. "Through it all," Nelson said, "Parcells talked to me as much as he could, always asked me how I was doing, my status, my workouts, was there anything he could do for me. Both his parents had passed away that year, and he was having a tough time. It was hard for Parcells to deal with somebody not indestructible. But he had more talks with me that year than anyone else on the team."

Every weekday, Nelson drove to Manhattan for his standing 9:45 A.M appointment, as methodical as ever, no shortcuts or detours, just Step A to Step B. Go for the radiation, kill the cancer cells; radiation therapy was a chore to be handled just like any other. "I saw my treatment as a form of training camp, and the doctor as my coach," Nelson recalled. "It was like going to work, only I got up in the morning and went to the hospital instead of the stadium. If the doctor told me what to do, I said, 'Okay, let's do it.'" Dig in. Plow through. Hold the line. "That regimented approach absolutely helped carry me through." All in all, he visited the radiologist 43 times.

"As an athlete, you're used to pushing yourself through tough situations," he said. "I knew I would be able to tolerate radiation because I was in good shape, and I was used to functioning when tired." All through radiation treatments, Nelson trained lightly, lifting dumbbells and riding a stationary bicycle. "I could still work out," he said. "But I had to take it easy and listen to my body."

Once, he went too far. He was lugging around some heavy rocks behind his house, putting in a swimming pool. He had slept poorly the previous two nights. Finished with his labors, he entered his home to take a shower. Suddenly, he vomited and felt lightheaded. He stumbled toward the kitchen for a glass of water to try to revive himself. Everything started to go dark on him. He leaned against the kitchen counter and blacked out, sliding down to the tiled floor. He awoke sprawled on his back, unaware of how he had gotten there. "I pushed myself too hard," he said. "It threw a scare into me and Heidi. If your body tells you to cool it, you should cool it."

Nelson played his emotions close to the vest. "I controlled my emotions because that's what I was taught to do," he said. "Sometimes I held in what I was feeling about the cancer. It went back to what Parcells told me about refusing to show that anything is going to get the better of you." This tight-lipped approach never sat well with Heidi. "I knew I would be able to deal with the disease, but Heidi did not know whether *she* could. I was letting none of my emotions out, and she was hungry for emotion from me at this point. But it was hard on Heidi. It was harder on her than on me."

"All he wanted to talk about," Heidi said, "was how long it was going to take him to get back to playing football."

"Heidi kept trying to kick me in the ass," Karl said. "She was telling me, 'Listen, forget about football. I'm tired of hearing about nothing but your return to football. I want to have a husband here and a father for our child.' She kept telling me that. But I just refused to listen."

Nelson finished radiation on December 9, 1987, having missed the entire football season. In the meantime, the Giants had drafted Eric Moore and John Elliot to replace him at right tackle. Nelson became a color commentator during Giant games on WNEW-Radio and hosted a pre-game talk show called "Tailgate Party."

To this point, he had fixated on the number Dr. Warren had cited, the 90 percent cure rate. But now he had second thoughts. "I always told the press, 'Oh I'm doing fine, I'm doing okay,'" he recalled. "I kind of trivialized the radiation treatments. But it was not all peaches and cream. I was in some denial. Maybe not so much denial as ignorance. I never had that fear because I knew nothing about it. I'd never gone through anything like that. I had no real personal experience with the disease. I'd never lost anyone to cancer. Then I realized, 'Hey, you never know. There *is* another 10 percent out there.'"

Around this time, Nelson met Jeff Blatnick. He, too, was a large fellow, 6 feet, 2 inches and 250 pounds, a super heavyweight Greco-Roman wrestler who had survived Hodgkin's disease to compete at the 1984 Los Angeles Olympics and come away with a gold medal. "It was a big plus for me to talk with somebody like Jeff," Nelson recalled. "He told me, 'You're gonna be fine, you're gonna be okay.' He gave me advice on what to expect, what I should do, what I should avoid. Listen to your body, stay positive—that kind of stuff. It was more reassurance than a pep talk, and it counted for a lot, especially coming from an Olympic gold medalist. It was great, and Jeff became a friend."

With the 1988 NFL season nine months ahead, Nelson contemplated his return to the Giants. He planned to play another three or four years in the league. "I'll be playing next season," he told anyone who asked.

"My goal was to get back to playing football again," he said. "That's what I wanted to do. Football gave me something important to shoot for. Nobody said it would be easy. But football was how I earned an income (he made $275,000 in his peak earning year). My attitude was, I've got to do everything I can to get back in uniform. All I wanted was get back to where I was."

❧ ❧ ❧

Everything had clicked for the New York Giants in 1986, including Karl Nelson, right tackle. In a game early in the season, for example, the Giants trailed the Minnesota Vikings by two points with less than a minute left. The Giants, facing a fourth-and-17, went for the first down. Unfortunately, Nelson had gotten whacked in the head on the previous down and was seeing double. He turned to fellow lineman Chris Godfrey. "Chris," he said, "I'm seeing double." Godfrey, deadpan, replied, "Just block the one on the right." Nelson followed this guidance on the next play, holding defenders away from quarterback Phil Simms long enough for him to complete a 22-yard pass. With only 12 seconds left, the Giants scored a field goal, pulling out a cliffhanger victory. "We had no right winning that football game," Nelson recalled. "It was fourth-and-17. No right at all."

The Giants won nine straight games that year by seven points or less. "Each game was a knockdown, drag-out war," he recalled, "and games like that, when you really get it going, are what football is all about. We were focused that year. We came together as a team and we always figured out how to win. That's the difference between a good team and a great team."

Each week Nelson thought, Okay, we won. Now let's think about next week. Let's win again so we can go on to the next game. He would start thinking about an upcoming game, picturing it in his mind, around Wednesday. By Friday, he would totally zone out. "Heidi and I would go out the Saturday night before a home game," he recalled. "And if we had candles on the table, she knew the night was done. I would just go into a trance staring at the candles. I had to focus on what I wanted to do on the field to make sure I was ready to play. She would talk to me and I would hear nothing." He blocked out thoughts he believed had no business being in his brain. Like the concept of losing.

That season, the Giants posted a 14–2 record. Nelson played every offensive down in every game, the only Giant to do so. With him at right tackle, Phil Simms finished the season ranked the fourth best quarterback in the NFL, completing 55.3 percent of his passes for 3,487 yards and 21 touchdowns. But Nelson best excelled at blocking for the run. Accordingly, the Giants called about 70 percent of all runs to go to the right, *his* side. Halfback Joe Morris carried the ball 341 times for 1,516 yards, averaging 4.4 yards a carry, and scored 14 touchdowns.

"I just went out and did my job," Nelson recounted.

In the 1986 playoffs, the Giants shifted into an even higher gear, first destroying the powerhouse San Francisco 49ers, 49–3, then trouncing the Washington Redskins, 17–0. "We always found a way to get it done that year," Nelson said. "If the offense was doing poorly in a game, the defense would pick it up. And if neither could do the job, the special teams would make the big play. We all believed in each other."

After shutting out the Redskins, the Giants celebrated quietly. "Getting to the Super Bowl was not going to be enough," Nelson said. "We wanted to win it."

In the Super Bowl the Giants fell behind the Denver Broncos, 10–9, in the second quarter. But Nelson still sniffed a victory in the offing. "It's funny," he said, "but when we went into the locker room at halftime, we all knew that even though we were losing, we had Denver exactly where we wanted. We told each other, 'We're not changing anything. Everything we're doing is working. We just have to put the ball in the end zone some more.' We were all very confident that we'd go out there and steamroll the Broncos in the second half, and that's exactly what we did."

Late in the third quarter, on a third down on the Denver 37-yard line, Nelson had his moment in the sun. Simms called a slant counter special, in which halfback Joe Morris would take a handoff and angle out behind Nelson. With the right tackle spearheading the attack, Morris barreled through the Denver line and rumbled into the secondary. As Nelson charged upfield, Morris rode on his hip, scanning for daylight. Then Nelson creamed a defensive back, slamming him flat on his behind, and freed the runner to motor along for a 12-yards gain to the Denver 25. The Giants then scored a touchdown, snatching the lead for the first time in the game.

The Giants won the 1987 Super Bowl, 39–20, with suffocating defense and a pulverizing offensive line. Thanks to Nelson and his fellow grunts, the team rushed for 136 yards, while the defense held Denver to only 52. More impressive still, the offensive line formed a hermetic membrane from behind which Phil Simms had time to spot receivers and fire away. The quarterback completed 22 of 25 passes and collected the Most Valuable Player Award for the game.

The Giants had generated so much momentum all season that after capturing the Super Bowl, Nelson wanted to keep going. "Standing on top of the mountain is nothing," he reflected. "It's getting there that's fun. We were on such a roll that all I could think was, 'Okay who do we play now?'"

❦ ❦ ❦

In April 1988, nine months after his diagnosis of cancer, Nelson arrived at Giants Stadium for the team's voluntary off-season training program. Dr. Wolf had pronounced his Hodgkin's in remission. Nelson still hoped to bash with the biggest and the best in the NFL, even though he found himself, as a result of surgery and radiation, easily winded and decidedly slower and weaker.

He worked out on a Cybex, a computerized resistance machine, executing bench presses and, of course, his trademark power cleans. He ran sprints, with a typical session consisting of eight 150-yard dashes, each separated by only a one-minute rest. By late spring, Nelson was working out five hours a day, four days a week, combining physical therapy, strength training and cardiovascular conditioning. Every day he performed power cleans with at least 135 pounds on the bar, cranking out six repetitions each for five sets.

"It's all coming together pretty good," Nelson said at the time. "I'm going to be ready. I'm going to play this year."

When the official Giants training camp opened in August, Coach Parcells decided to push Nelson hard, cutting him no slack. "Everyone is giving Karl Nelson sympathy but me," Parcells said. The coach instructed his left defensive ends George Martin and Eric Dorsey to waylay Nelson at every opportunity in the twice-a-day practices. "His doctors told me I could push him, so I do," Parcells said during the summer camp. "Do you think I like yelling at him? He's a great kid, and he's got every excuse in the book for not making it back to the team. But he's just got to do it. He's working hard, but nobody gets gold medals for trying hard. You're *supposed* to try hard. You win gold medals for getting it done."

Nelson still had a special camaraderie with the other grunts.

Godfrey, Oates, Ard, and Benson warmly welcomed him back to the team. He could always count on the other grunts to come through.

Nelson played in an exhibition game against the New York Jets, his first contest in a year. He stayed in at right tackle for about 40 plays, keeping defensive end Mark Gastineau from a single tackle or sack. "I'm encouraged," Parcells said.

Nelson regained his starting spot at right tackle for the September 5 season opener against the Washington Redskins at the Meadowlands, the game featured on the WABC-TV "Monday Night Football" telecast. Nelson quickly realized that his timing and his rhythm were off more than a beat. "My body refused to do what I asked it to do," he recalled. "I was too excited to play well, just out of control."

But Karl Nelson had at least come back, come back after two major surgeries and 43 radiation treatments, to play right tackle in the NFL and push and shove with the big boys. He had dug in, plowed through and held the line. He started the next game, too, against the 49ers. But then he tore ligaments in his right ankle and sat out the next seven weeks. Late in the season, Nelson played again, facing the New York Jets, with a playoff berth at stake. He shuttled in and out of the lineup as Parcells deployed him specially for third-down-and-short yardage, plays that exploited his specialty for run-blocking. The team finished the season with nine wins, seven losses.

On December 14, 1988, Nelson saw Dr. Wolf for a three-month checkup, believing himself to be out of the woods. But Wolf found a lump on his left side, next to his collarbone. Nelson thought the growth might be a swollen gland, an inconsequential thyroid problem. The Hodgkin's had recurred, and Wolf took out the lump. Karl went home to tell the news to Heidi, who was pregnant with a second Nelson child, her due date only two weeks away. "It's back," he told her. "You've got to be kidding," she responded.

The next week, Heidi gave birth to a second daughter, Lyndsay.

Now came chemotherapy for her husband. As with radiation, Nelson regarded chemo as a facsimile of training camp, with his oncologist acting as coach. The drug therapy, taken both orally and intravenously, required 28-day cycles for the next six months. "Chemotherapy is the worst nightmare you'll ever go through in your entire life," Nelson said. "Chemo was 10 times worse than radiation. I had tubes and catheters coming out of my body for seven months. My face was bloated. It was impossible for me to sleep. After I lost my hair, I wore a wig. If I felt hot at home, I would ask my 2-year-old daughter, 'Brittany, do you mind if I take off my hair?' And she would say, 'No, Daddy, that's okay.'"

"It's a bitch not being in charge of your life," he said. "Cancer rules you. It limits how you're going to feel, what you can do, where you can go. When my white blood cell count was low and my temperature was high, I had to be quarantined for several days a month to avoid infection. But you have to realize that it's not the end of the world. I told myself I was not going to die from this. I never felt my life was threatened. I always felt positive about all my treatments. I believe a positive attitude will help you get through. You need to go on and try to make your life as normal as possible.

"But I was scared," he said. "The second time around with cancer, I was definitely scared. But I was confident-scared. It goes back to that idea of using fear as a positive, as a motivator. I took that idea from football so I could control my emotions and my fear during chemo. It helped me."

He finished the treatments in July 1989 and once again eyed a comeback bid. In the locker room, an atmosphere of solemnity surrounded Nelson. His presence induced a sobriety that veteran linebacker Harry Carson wanted to shatter. "Hey, Karl," he would yell cheerfully across the locker room. "How's your chemo going?"

But Nelson sat out the 1989 season, and by then he knew the story. He had dug in. He had plowed through. He had held the line. He had come back from the thoracotomy and the splenectomy and the laparotomy and the 43 radiation treatments. He had come back to wear jersey number 63 for the Giants a few more games, and that was going to be it. Step A to Step B, from athlete to ex-athlete. The struggle had taken everything out of him, and now, the chemo further weakening him, his shoulders and knees bothering him, too, he had nothing left. He had played his last game.

On December 13, the 29-year-old went into the media room at Giants Stadium for a press conference and announced his retirement. "I'm no longer going to try to come back," Nelson told reporters. "I played less than I wanted to last year, and not as well as I wanted to. After I hurt my ankle, I never got going, never felt like the same player. It's an accumulation of problems, mainly the cancer, but also arthritis in my knee and shoulder. I've accomplished about everything a football player could want, including a win in the Super Bowl. Now it's time for me to get on with my life... outside football."

He thanked the Giants and the media, and left the podium.

Nelson now has a full-time job as a financial adviser for National Insurance Associates in Paramus, New Jersey, handling mostly pensions and employee benefits. He also still broadcasts Giants games on radio. He is closely involved with Tomorrow's Children Fund, an organization that supports children afflicted with cancer. "I can tell a kid I've gone through what he's gone through," he said. No longer in need of power cleans, he has trimmed down to 235 pounds. Every six months he goes for checkups, and shows no sign of a recurrence. He feels healthy except that he catches colds easily, and the bottoms of his feet constantly feel asleep, a side effect of the chemotherapy.

He is left now with the vivid physical mementos of his cancer. His chest still shows the 16 black-dye pinpoints from radiotherapy. An 11-inch scar wraps around the right side of his ribs to his spine, and a thick, pink, 12-inch stripe divides his stomach in half, from breastbone to navel.

"I never asked, 'Why me?'" he said. "I just pushed ahead. I thought, 'All right, this is happening. Now, what do I have to do to get better?'

"Truth is, I might not have handled cancer as well without my being an athlete. In football, you learn to set a goal, to be persistent, to be dedicated. Football kept me going all through my cancer. I just wanted more than anything to get back to playing. I knew if I could get back to football, I would be okay. And once I did, I was."

Chapter 5

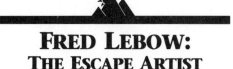

FRED LEBOW:
THE ESCAPE ARTIST

On a Tuesday night in late February 1990, Fred Lebow lay in Mount Sinai Medical Center in upper Manhattan, alone, crying for the first time in more than 50 years. He had found out earlier in the day that he had a rare cancer of the brain. His family and friends had visited and left, and now he was free to cry without an audience. A malignant tumor had grown in the left frontal lobe of his skull, and the doctor had told him that he probably had only three months left to live, maybe six.

But Lebow was not crying about the disease that now threatened to kill him. No, he was weeping about an incident that had occurred more than 50 years earlier, back in his native country of Rumania. He had long since forgotten about the episode, only to realize that he had carried the memory with him through half a century and across the Atlantic Ocean to America.

Alone in his hospital room, Lebow suspected that at some point in his life he had committed a wrong, a grievous sin that had tainted his soul and spurred the tumor. He wanted to recall his mistakes and come clean. Then something had stabbed him in the heart, creating an ache of remorse and guilt, and brought on tears. And now, in the flickering cinema of recollection, he vaguely remembered why he was crying, why, indeed, he had broken down with shame as a bony little boy on a European city street in 1938, before World War II scattered his family around the globe.

It was the chick. It was definitely the chick.

Lebow seldom indulged in introspection. Like many an entrepreneur, he sallied forth on instinct and operated in fast-forward. He would move on to the next deal, almost never dwelling on mistakes or second-guessing himself. That was how he had established an empire. That was how he had become president of the New York Road Runners Club and created an internationally renowned event known as the New York City Marathon. Besides,

Lebow himself was a marathoner. He had completed no fewer than 68 marathons, and in the marathon you never look back. What counts is not the previous mile covered but the next step taken.

But this was different. This was not business. This was cancer of the brain. So Lebow felt forced to look back and ask himself what terrible wrong had gnawed at him for so many years. Then the images of light and shadow swirling in his memory slowly crystallized.

"At first I denied to myself that I had cancer," Lebow recalled. "I felt so nervous and upset the day I heard the diagnosis that I hardly even realized what the doctor had said. I kept thinking, Probably someone has made a mistake, a serious mistake. I felt I was healthy. I kept saying to the doctor, 'I'm healthy. I've never had even a headache or dizziness, forget about a disease.' I had no symptoms of a cancerous tumor. So I denied it. I ignored the prognosis—just forgot about it.

"But when you're in the hospital, you have lots of time to think," he said. "It was the first time I had had this kind of oasis. I was able to think about myself in depth. My mind played games with me, and I decided that the physician was right—that I *would* last only three to six more months. I felt sorry for myself. That night in Mount Sinai I believed I would not make it. I was ready to join the world of dead people. Still, I thought it should have waited another 40 years to happen, this cancer. Why me? Why now? I wanted to find out. I needed to know. Maybe, I thought, it was something I had done. Maybe God was punishing me for misbehaving. And I began looking through my life.

"Suddenly I wanted to confess my sins. I thought about my days smuggling diamonds as a boy in Europe. I thought about the women I had lived with. I asked myself, had I treated those women right? Was I abusive? It seemed that my only sin was in not being married. But then I remembered the incident about the chick."

Lebow was ensconced in his office, stockinged feet propped on his desk. Lean and bearded, with pale blue eyes and thinning hair, he tilted back in his chair, looking upward in a trance of memory. An overhead fan whirred away above his desk. He had asked his secretary to hold all calls. In a soft, raspy voice, with a heavy accent that harks back to his Eastern European heritage, he told the story of why he cried.

"I remembered being only six years old, in Rumania, before World War II," he said. "I was walking on a road with my friends. I was going from my house to the main section of town, only two blocks. It was a city street, but it had a country atmosphere. A farmer went by in the road, and he was followed by a mother hen with a dozen chicks behind her. The chicks toddled along in a line, all small and yellow and fuzzy. I'd always loved those little chickies and wanted one as my pet. So I scooped up the last chick in my palm and ran down the road, back to my house. I decided that my pet goat should have a companion and that I would keep the chick in the backyard.

"I remembered I sat that night on a stool in front of my house. It was dark. And from inside I heard the neighbor who owned the chickens tell my father I had stolen the chick. I had left my cap on the street early that day, and he found out it was me and told my father. My parents knew and gave back the chick and never punished me, and I never found out what happened to the chick. I felt so ashamed that I cried. And that was what had bothered me for more than 50 years. It was the only bad deed I could remember. And after my diagnosis at Mount Sinai, I cried for the first time since the incident. Then I thought, So this is what I've worried about all these years—that I stole a chick."

He had stolen a chick, and now cancer threatened to steal his life. Hardly a quid pro quo.

"I went through so much in that one restless evening in the hospital," Lebow said. "It lasted only about two hours, all this remembering, but it felt like the longest night of my life. I realized I was not so bad after all. I was a pretty good guy. I had never insulted or hit anyone. I had treated women well. I had not known this about myself—that I was okay. I had not appreciated myself as a man. And I stopped crying. My last thought before I fell asleep was about the chick. I realized I had nothing to be sorry about anymore. I had forgiven myself, and it was like a revelation. I woke at seven the next morning feeling great, ready to fight my cancer."

❦ ❦ ❦

In late 1989, several months before the doctor delivered his diagnosis, Fred Lebow began, ever so subtly, to change. Around the offices at the New York Road Runners Club, his brisk gait slowed. He trod along unsure of his step, his arms occasionally groping for the nearest support, as if any minute he might lose his balance and keel over. He grew absent-minded and forgetful, suddenly seemed distant and older than his 57 years.

Lebow would lay down his glasses on his desk and two minutes later ask, "Whose glasses are those?"

"Those are yours, Fred," Brian Crawford, a close friend since 1957 and an administrator at the club, would point out.

"Oh. Do I wear glasses?"

"Of course you do, Fred."

"No, they're not my glasses. I never wore glasses."

"Yes, Fred, believe me, you wear glasses and those are your glasses."

Lebow also forgot names and faces. In February 1990, he attended the annual awards banquet for the New York Road Runners Club. Speaking from the podium, Lebow announced an award winner. Then two minutes later, he introduced another honoree, but mistakenly gave the same name as before. "It was weird," Lebow recalled. "I would look right at people I knew and forget who they were."

More than a few staff members at the club noticed that Lebow seemed different from before. Out of it. Almost lost. Sandy Sislowitz, a social psychologist and volunteer at the club, called Crawford. "Something is wrong with Fred," Sislowitz said. Crawford replied, "I know. We have to do something."

"For at least a couple of weeks, Fred did not seem well," Crawford recalled. "Some people here at the club suspected he might have become depressed or had a stroke. I remember that one day Fred decided, out of the blue, to call his brothers who live in Israel and Montreal. Now, Fred never called his brothers. So afterwards I asked him why he had called. He just said he thought he should. It was as if it had dawned on him that something might be wrong with him. He just felt, at that moment, that he should be closer to his family."

The last straw came on a Sunday in late February. Crawford tagged along with Lebow on a visit to Westchester, New York, to see Lebow's sister, Sarah Katz. "I remember that after the visit, we drove back to his apartment building on the Upper East Side of Manhattan," Crawford said. "Fred got out of the car and leaned onto the window and said to me, 'Good night, old friend.' He had never said anything like that to me before."

Crawford looked at his friend of more than 30 years standing beside the car, smiling. He told Lebow he should see a doctor. But Crawford pretended the visit should revolve around his troublesome left knee rather than all the other disturbing symptoms that had recently come to light. Lebow mumbled okay. That night Crawford called Dr. Norbert Sander to let him know that Fred would visit him for an appointment the next day, ostensibly about his knee. But Crawford made plain to Sander that he believed Lebow should receive a complete work-up. Moments later, Crawford faxed a message to the New York Road Runners Club. He wanted Lebow to see the fax as soon as he got to the office the next morning. The fax contained only one word: DOCTOR.

The next day Lebow saw the fax and promptly went to see Dr. Sander, a 1974 winner of the New York City Marathon, at New Rochelle Hospital in Westchester. Dr. Sander referred him to Dr. Seymour Gendelman, a neurologist at Mount Sinai Medical Center in Manhattan. Dr. Gendelman examined Lebow and subjected him to several tests, including a magnetic resonance imaging procedure. After he reviewed the test results, he detected a growth in Lebow's head. He scheduled a biopsy to identify the mass. In the process, he cut through the side of his skull and withdrew a tissue specimen for a pathologist to evaluate.

A day later, Dr. Gendelman had diagnosed the problem: Lebow had a malignant tumor in his brain approximately the size of a tennis ball (or so it seemed because of all the swollen tissue surrounding it). The doctor had found a central nervous system lymphoma, a form of cancer that typically develops in the chest, stomach, and other regions of the body, but rarely occurs in so sensitive a precinct as the brain.

Central nervous system cancers, wherever they materialize, are rare, accounting for only about one in every 75 malignancies. According to the American Cancer Society, brain cancer in general causes only about one in every 50 cancer deaths and claimed nearly 11,000 lives in 1988, the last year for which reliable statistics are available. (For reasons still undetermined, male patients with brain cancer outnumber females approximately three to two.) In 1958, only 30 years earlier, roughly twice as many died of the disease. Until a few decades ago, the standard treatment was radiation therapy alone. The prognosis for brain cancer patients remained poor.

Dr. Gendelman told Lebow that unless the growth shrank—drastically and fast—he was facing death.

☙ ☙ ☙

Fischel Leibowitz was born in western Rumania, in the small Transylvanian town of Arad, 10 miles from Hungary and 40 from Yugoslavia. He was the second youngest of seven children in a devout Orthodox Jewish family. His father was a wholesale produce distributor. When the Nazis occupied Arad, his father was forced to give up his business and sent to a work camp, where he was ordered to wear a yellow star stigmatizing him as a Jew. Later the young boy would learn that the Nazis had murdered his grandparents, uncles, aunts, and cousins in Hungary and Czechoslovakia.

In 1945, in the immediate aftermath of World War II, the Russian Communists seized Rumania. The Liebowitz family split up and escaped. Leibowitz, then 13, fled his homeland forever. He ran in the dark and the cold, through gunfire and bombing, past slain soldiers and dying horses, to a Bulgarian village, where sympathizers concealed him in a room for two days. Then he hopped onto a train and hid in a baggage compartment, thus slipping into Czechoslovakia. From there the boy migrated to Holland, along with thousands of other refugees, then headed north to England and Dublin, jumping freight cars for free, anonymous passage to freedom.

Leibowitz lived like a fugitive all through his teenage years. By the age of 16, he was smuggling sugar from one country to another, always selling to the highest bidder. Soon he would hire himself out as a courier who, for a hefty fee, would sneak across borders smuggling diamonds packaged in prophylactics. In this exodus from the persecution of Nazis and Communists, he learned a lesson in the survival of crisis, for such an ordeal might have traumatized a less hardy individual. The brush with totalitarian regimes forever stamped him, defined him, as an escape artist, a hustler, an opportunist, quick on his feet and ever-ready to cut a deal, whether with border patrols, corporate sponsors, or brain cancer. "As a young boy, I was always on the lookout for someone chasing me," Lebow recalled. For the next 15 years, he lost contact with his family and Judaism.

In 1951, he arrived in the United States, first in Kansas City, then in Cleveland, where he eventually sold TV sets wholesale and ran an improvisational theater and roomed with Brian Crawford. In the mid-1960s, Fischel Liebowitz—now reincarnated, if not reconstituted, as Fred Lebow, a fully assimilated U.S. citizen—settled in Brooklyn, then Manhattan, renting a $69-a-month apartment on East 53rd Street with Crawford. He attended classes at the New York Fashion Institute and quickly became a specialist in knockoffs in the garment district.

He went into his office early in the morning, left late at night, and never missed a day. His modus operandi was to analyze an original designer garment worth, say, $200. Then he would tinker with the elements of its composition to make it his own. For example, he would transform a 14-ounce fabric to 12-ounce, reduce the six buttons to five, convert the real pockets to fake, and remove the lining. He would then order the garment manufactured in Hong Kong or Italy and market the duplicated item, give or take a few fine points, not for $200 or even $100, but merely $50. Lebow sold these low-cost polyester copies of designer fashions and within a few years amassed a fortune.

Lebow played tennis two or three times a week as a sideline, always against his pal Crawford. Although Lebow competed intensely, chasing down every shot, he always lost these games, much to his chagrin. By 1969, he lapsed into such a funk over this losing streak, and his own general incompetence in the sport, that he considered seeking guidance from a psychiatrist. A tennis coach advised Lebow that he would probably perform better on the courts if he developed more strength and stamina. So Lebow hoisted weights for a few weeks, until he grew bored with this regimen and quit. A physical trainer then suggested Lebow take a crack at running to enhance his endurance. He recommended, in particular, the path around the reservoir in the middle of Central Park.

So it was that Lebow ventured out on his first run, with his buddy Crawford loping along as a partner. Lebow at this point wanted only to condition his heart, lungs, and legs, the better to bird-dog shots on the tennis court. Still, ever the competitor, especially against Crawford, Lebow wagered his pal that he would complete the 1.5-mile loop first. Crawford accepted the bet, but, after running only one mile, he was so winded that he had to stop. Meanwhile, Lebow kept going and finished the course, cashing in on the modest gamble.

But in the 10 minutes or so that Lebow had galloped along this path in the park, he discovered that running gave him the keenest joy. He relished the feel of the earth passing quickly under his feet, the sweat pouring down his brow and neck, the accelerated pounding of his heart. Never again would he play tennis.

❧ ❧ ❧

Lebow's younger sister Sarah took the news about his cancer hardest. Of all the other brothers and sisters in the Liebowitz clan, Sarah was the sibling closest to Fred, and the most nakedly emotional as well. The doctor told her point-blank that her brother had a brain tumor and probably only three to six months to live. After hearing this message, Sarah rode in a car with Crawford back to her Westchester home, sobbing and babbling and hysterical. "How could this happen?" she wailed. "How could this happen to Fred of all people? He's an athlete." Crawford tried to console her, to little avail.

"I was shattered to hear about the lymphoma," Sarah recalled. "I thought, How can this be? We had never had cancer in our family before. It was impossible to believe. Incredible. Fred was suddenly in the intensive care unit at Mount Sinai, and the doctors gave him a 50-50 chance of survival, and I could not sleep. But I knew he would live. My family, we're fighters."

Within a week of his arrival at Mount Sinai, Lebow received visits from all his brothers and sisters. Sarah came in from Westchester, Simcha from Brooklyn, Morris from Cleveland, Michael from Chicago, and Schlomo from Tel Aviv. "It was the first time in my life my family came together to the same place to spend time as brothers and sisters," Lebow recalled. "Before I got sick, I never saw family at all. I had thought: Family? Brothers and sisters? Who cares? I saw my brothers and sisters, individually, only once every year or two. But now I realized how much they cared about me. And I realized how much I cared, too."

Friends, too, turned out by the dozens. Brian Crawford gravitated to the hospital room, along with Allan Steinfeld, the executive vice president of the New York Road Runners Club; and long-time friend Richard Traum, president of the Achilles Club for disabled runners, who himself had an artificial leg. Girlfriend Heather Rose Dominic, a lovely, doe-eyed 23-year-old actress, stopped in to see the ailing marathoner; and former girlfriends, such as author and *New Yorker* writer Connie Bruck, also came by. Along with club staffers and other well-wishers were the elite runners of the previous two decades, all of whom had competed either in the New York City Marathon or other events held by the New York Road Runners Club. Bill Rodgers, who won the New York City Marathon four times, was there, and so was Joan Benoit-Samuelson, a female marathon Olympic gold medalist. Middle-distance Olympian Mary Decker Slaney and Eamonn Coghlan, former holder of the indoor mile record, showed up.

One nurse, witnessing this outpouring of sympathy and the parade of girlfriends, active and retired, one afternoon turned to Sarah in the hospital corridor and said in reference to Lebow, "I have no idea who he is, but he must be a movie star, because so many gorgeous girls have come to see him."

Lebow admirers, concerned about not only his spirits but also his health, sent the patient purported cure-alls for cancer. The drawers and closets in his hospital room and at the club quickly spilled over with hundreds of letters recommending all manner of panaceas, at least 50 books offering quick fixes, not to mention a raft of cans, jars, and tubes, all containing miracle powders, ointments, gels, and the like (including a drink of wheat grass), each one a potential nostrum for the scourges of cancer.

Bouquet after bouquet arrived in the hospital room. Roses and tulips, daffodils and chrysanthemums—a rainbow profusion of flowers and plants perfuming the otherwise antiseptic air of Mount Sinai. Lebow loyalists dispatched so many flowers that the nurses had to mount an extra shelf on the wall in his room, and then haul in an extra table, and even that was not enough.

Richard Traum, who holds a doctorate in behavioral sciences and has known Lebow since 1975, recalled the scene in the hospital: "Fred received so many calls and visitors that he needed someone to manage it all. We had to field more than a hundred calls a day, including many from the media. Thousands of people contacted him with encouragement. Fred was surprised and overwhelmed by all the love and affection he received. He never knew people felt so strongly about him, and the attention made him feel important. For the first time in his life he became reflective. He realized he had really accomplished something with his life." Said Sarah, "I've never seen a man more loved. So much love. I believe Fred benefited from all the love people poured out to him. It made him feel good. It strengthened him. And he would need that strength."

❦ ❦ ❦

From 1969 on, Lebow ran around the reservoir in Central Park at every opportunity, always by himself (because Crawford would have difficulty keeping up with him). He developed a habit of taking off time from his job as a garment consultant in the middle of the day to duck out for an invigorating run. One day, Lebow happened to chat with a fellow jogger, a member of the New York Road Runners Club, who mentioned that he ran in local road races and told Lebow of an upcoming five-mile race around Yankee Stadium. Eager to express his competitive spirit in a formal setting, Lebow said, "I would like to try that."

Lebow immediately registered for his inaugural race. Facing several dozen competitors, he circumvented the Bronx landmark 11 times and finished second to last. (To this day, he claims that if he had come in last, he would have dropped the sport for good.) Despite this lackluster performance, he found the run exhilarating. He shelled out $3 for membership privileges in the New York Road Runners Club.

Lebow entered all the races the club scheduled over the next few months, mostly cross-country affairs, and whipped himself into shape. In March 1970, the club held its annual Cherry Tree Marathon in the Bronx, and Lebow declared himself fit for a maiden effort in the 26-mile, 385-yard event. As it turned out, he clocked a highly respectable time: 4:09, averaging about nine minutes per mile.

But he was dismayed to notice that the race had no spectators along its circuitous route through the Bronx. Besides this pronounced lack of public interest, the runners encountered more than a few hurdles before reaching the finish line. The contestants had to navigate roadways with an often-menacing presence of cars, buses, and cabs, all well-schooled in the New York City style of kamikaze driving. The streets of the Bronx, bleak with burnt-out tenements, were lined with teenagers who, evidently lacking better opportunities for recreation than target practice, pelted passing runners with stones.

After the race, Lebow found himself musing about his daily runs through Central Park. Its roads were wide and smooth, virtually free of potholes and vehicles, and runners could coast in relative safety and pastoral quiet through its dales and meadows, past the birds and squirrels and trees. He thought, Why not a marathon in Central Park?

Wasting no time, he proposed the idea to the board of directors at the New York Road Runners Club. "He was the one who thought of running the first marathon through Central Park," said Brian Crawford. "But all the board members hesitated—Fred really had a lot of opposition. People thought, You're crazy if you want to let people wearing nothing but underwear run through the park. But Fred always knew what he wanted."

Burly and tanned, with an easy smile and blue eyes, Crawford sat in his windowless office decked out in blue jeans, baseball cap, and sneakers, and recounted the early days at the club with Lebow. "I remember when Fred and I first met with the board of directors," Crawford said. "They said, 'A marathon in Central Park! What happens if you lose money on the deal?' Fred said, 'That's okay. We'll put up the money. Right, Brian?' He looked at me, and we both knew we had no money. But I just nodded as if it was okay."

"Fred never had any doubts about a marathon in Central Park," Crawford reflected. "Whatever he wanted done, he thought he could do. He was a big-picture guy. He never wanted to bother with the details. He always let someone else deal with details, and he never took no for an answer. Or he might accept no for an answer, but then he went ahead and did whatever he wanted anyway. He would let you think he liked your idea, and then he would do what he wanted. I remember we once had a meeting to discuss which color of T-shirt to order for the first marathon, and everyone at the club said, 'Let's get white ones.' And Fred said, 'Well, I like orange T-shirts.' And they said, 'Oh, no, we'll have to get the white ones.' And Fred said, 'Okay.' And then, after the meeting, he said to me, 'Brian, go ahead and order the orange T-shirts.'"

In 1970, marathons were still consigned to the outskirts of legitimate athletics, its participants maligned as nerds, nuts, fanatics, freaks, pseudo-athletes, and worse. In this climate, the New York Road Runners Club appointed Fred Lebow to be director of the first marathon in Central Park. From the kitchen table in his apartment, Lebow mapped out a labyrinthian four-lap circuit.

The 1970 New York City Marathon in Central Park enlisted 126 runners, of whom 72 finished (including Lebow, with a 4:12, good for 44th place). Several hundred curious New Yorkers stood along the route and looked on. A modest success, all in all, but a success nevertheless. No run-ins with cabs, potholes, or rock-brandishing teenagers.

Lebow, hardly satisfied to watch others run and never inclined to go halfway with anything, competed in about one marathon a month all through 1970. That year he ran in 13 marathons, including races in Paris, Oslo, Stockholm, and Syracuse, New York, (where he posted a personal best of 3:19, averaging about eight minutes per mile).

In 1972, on the thrust of his enterprise and vision, Lebow was promoted to president of the New York Road Runners Club. The organization had 270 members at the time. In 1975 he rented a few small, cramped rooms as an office at the West Side YMCA. Nobody had an inkling that under his stewardship, this embryo known as the New York City Marathon would grow to be the biggest and best known event of its kind in the world.

❧ ❧ ❧

Chemotherapy under Dr. Gendelman at Mount Sinai consisted of a combination of cyclophosphamide, vincristine, and adriamycin. Lebow withstood the drug treatments without complaint.

"Fred never said anything negative about his cancer," Crawford recalled. "Never said, 'This is terrible.' Never questioned the diagnosis, never expressed self-pity. On a couple of occasions, he seemed to want to talk about the cancer, but then we would get onto another subject. It was like we had an agreement. We both knew he had a disease, but we never talked about it. We never really discussed it, because he said, 'I'm going to get better,' and he felt he had nothing to discuss. His attitude was that the cancer was just a little sickness. He would say, 'I'll get through this.' He always acted as if everything would stay normal and he would keep going as he had before. It was understood that after he was in the hospital, he would come back to run the club. Nothing was going to stop him.

"But it was a tough time for Fred. And he started to give in. During the chemotherapy he had his doubts. He lost his hair and seemed weaker. He told me we should make Allan Steinfeld president of the club. I said, 'Why should we? Why should we talk about it now? First you'll get out of the hospital and then we'll see.' I never said any specific words of support or encouragement to Fred. If I helped him at all, it was by acting as if we would go on the same as before."

Sarah, in frequent visits to his bedside, found her brother ready to face the challenges of cancer. "Fred always acted strong in front of me," she said, "and never felt sorry for himself. I think that made a difference for him. He seemed very relaxed. Fred knows life is something very precious that God gives you, and you are responsible for it. He believes in positive thinking. He would always turn negative into positive. I would tell him that his life was so much more exciting than mine, but he would tell me that my visits to him were the most exciting event of his day."

"He was always looking to the future," Sarah said. "Planning. He seemed to want to put everything in order. He believed that if he put everything in order—such as his relationship with all his brothers and sisters—he could also put his health in order. The first time he spoke about his cancer, he said that whatever happens, happens. He said, 'I'm very happy. I have accomplished a lot and I've had a wonderful life.' For a moment he sounded like he was ready to leave us. I said, 'Fred, what about us?' meaning his brothers and sisters. He just smiled, and we never spoke of the problem again."

One morning at Mount Sinai, Lebow felt unusually adventurous, even for him. Unknown to the doctors and nurses, he rolled out of bed, walked down a hallway, and went through a door. He found himself, much to his surprise, standing on a rooftop terrace, with all of upper Manhattan spread out below. The March air felt chilly and bracing against his skin, and he decided to walk around. He had gone several weeks without any exercise, let alone a run, and he missed his daily dose of physical exertion.

He walked one lap around the terrace, then another. The rooftop was only about 50 feet long and 30 feet wide, probably less than 50 yards all around. As Lebow walked his laps, cranking out step after step, he calculated that to cover a mile, he would need to go around the terrace 67 times. Not 65 or 70. And so, with yet another course mapped out, Lebow walked laps on the roof the next day and the day after. Still cautious about his condition, he chose to walk rather than run. First he registered a mile, then a mile-and-a-half, then two. Finally, Lebow told Dr. Gendelman about his increasingly brisk forays into the daylight. The doctor, rather than calling him to task for this self-therapy, complimented him on his commitment to recovery and encouraged him to keep at it.

"If you feel like running," Dr. Gendelman said, "then run."

Eventually, Lebow started to run on the roof. He plodded round and round, 67 laps to the mile, no more and no less. Never before had he needed nearly so many circuits to run a mile. But he kept going because even during exposure to chemo, he felt more natural running on a rooftop than reclining in bed all day as nurses checked his chart. The running gave Lebow a lifeline. "Fred had to get in his run," Crawford said. "He was very strict about putting the miles down in his log." On each outing, Lebow lifted his feet higher and lengthened his stride, the ground moving faster under his feet and his heart pounding harder. Though still trudging, he felt the same joy as he had 20 years earlier racing Crawford for money. Only now, the stakes were much higher.

🐞 🐞 🐞

Every morning in the early 1970s, Lebow ran roughly a mile from his Manhattan apartment on East 72nd Street between First and Second Avenues to his office at the New York Road Runners Club and then headed into Central Park to cover another mile or two. He preferred to run around the reservoir because the footing was solid and the loops were easy to time and the workout took long enough to feel rigorous. He always ran alone.

While running, he would engage in his most creative thinking of the day. He developed a habit, rather eccentric by most standards, but certainly fruitful: every time an idea came to him during a run, he would grab a twig and scratch a key word in the dirt along the pathway. The only problem was that whenever he went back to the spot to read the inscribed memo to himself, the words were already rubbed away. Lebow took another tack: he would return to his desk with the twig as a mnemonic device. He soon discovered that looking at the twig restored the idea to his mind.

One idea Lebow scribbled in the soil was for a marathon that would extend beyond the environs of Central Park and branch out into all the reaches of New York City, a race that would course through the arteries of all five boroughs of Manhattan, Brooklyn, Queens, the Bronx, and Staten Island. The Central Park event had drawn enough runners and sponsors and media interest to warrant expansion into an occasion of citywide civic significance, Lebow believed. Why not? he thought. Why not a five-borough marathon?

Once again, board members at the New York Road Runners Club considered the idea impossible, if not lunatic. It would be a nightmare of red tape and logistics, they claimed. Five boroughs? Each was a municipality unto itself, rife with rules and regulations. But once again, Lebow—largely by force of conviction—prevailed. In 1976, the club organized the first five-borough New York City Marathon. The race snaked from Staten Island to Brooklyn, along Fourth Avenue across the Pulaski Bridge into Queens, over the Queensboro Bridge and north on First Avenue, across the Willis Avenue Bridge into the Bronx, back over the Madison Avenue Bridge into Manhattan, and down along the spine of Central Park to the finish line.

And in 1977, as a direct consequence of this success, New York City declared January 12 to be Fred Lebow Day. Lebow quit the garment industry to devote himself full-time to the fortunes of the club. In 1981, the New York Road Runners Club bought a building on East 89th Street, just a few doors away from Fifth Avenue and less than 100 yards from Central Park, to serve as its headquarters. Designated the International Running Center, the 19th-century stone mansion had six floors with 40 rooms. Cost: $1.3 million. Lebow had graduated from the kitchen table in his apartment space.The émigré from Arad had officially attained VIP status in the United States.

But what seems rather imperial from the outside is a no-frills proposition inside. The walls throughout the structure are smudged with fingerprints, paint on the doors is peeling, and the carpeting is stained. Lebow installed his office on the fourth floor, with a window overlooking an air shaft, hardly a presidential view. With runners always milling about in the lobby, whether to sign entry blanks for races or check the bulletin board messages for partners or to pick up fliers and schedules, the atmosphere is collegiate, like that of a university for runners. Here enthusiasts young and old, large and small, rich and poor, swift and slow, converge as comrades of equal stature, often sweating and gasping as they chat about how many miles they ran that day and how wonderful (or lousy) they felt doing it.

Lebow himself set the style for the club, with his casual, soft-spoken demeanor, though he was occasionally accused of being aloof and behaving like a taskmaster. From the start, he lived a monastic life, especially for the head of an organization whose power and popularity were growing so fast. He rented a small apartment and had no car. He never took cabs and ate only two light, inexpensive meals a day. He survived on several thousand dollars a year. Race sponsors and patrons provided all his meals and trips, and he wore only complementary running clothes. He donned these freebie get-ups—customarily baggy warm-up pants, sweat socks, T-shirts, running shoes, Italian-style bicycling caps—because it was his policy to wear only what was given him. Never one to stand on ceremony, he wore the outfits everywhere—the office, airplanes, business trips, even swanky restaurants. He looked as if any minute he might break into a run, and sometimes he would.

The compulsion to make tracks overtook Lebow often indeed. He maintained his routine of covering three or four miles a day in Central Park, sometimes logging his distances in both the morning and evening of the same day, and only once in a while would he skip a workout. On weekends, true to form, he would set out for longer runs of 15 or 20 miles to prime himself for races. All along, he ran not only for fun but also for competition. He entered approximately one marathon a month through the 1970s and finished every one. He raced in marathons in Boston, London, Shanghai (as a guest of the Chinese government), and Moscow.

Lebow liked to wax rhapsodic about long-distance running. "Running is the only sport of its kind," he would say. "It's just you. You run without skis attached to your legs, without a rope around your waist, without a helmet on your head, without any equipment at all. Running is the oldest sport of all, and the most natural. It should be accepted not just as a sport but as a lifestyle. Doctors should prescribe exercise. People should run to work, and companies should put in showers for employees. Running should become second nature, like brushing your teeth."

But never in all those years would he run in the five-borough New York City Marathon. He was too busy organizing the event—lining up sponsors, securing municipal permits, clearing the route. "When I'm in the lead car and we're approaching the finish line," Lebow said in 1982, "I always wish I were running instead. So one of these days I'm just going to do it. I'm going to run in our own New York Marathon."

❧ ❧ ❧

In April 1990 Lebow transferred to Memorial Sloan-Kettering Cancer Center and added radiation treatments to his chemo regimen. There, he came under the care of attending neurologist Dr. Lisa M. DeAngelis. All well and good, except that he now found himself without access to a proper running facility. So one day, he went out into the halls at Memorial to count the tiles. Nobody witnessing this act had a clue about what he was doing. Down the hall he went, tile by tile, as methodical as an actuary computing a life span. He marked off a circuit of about 200 yards, designing yet another impromptu, makeshift hospital course, and commenced to walk laps, fast, almost as if race walking. Dr. DeAngelis, like Dr. Gendelman, endorsed his verve and independence.

Lebow was convinced, as he made his rounds at Memorial, that if he could sustain this program, other cancer patients on the floor could follow suit. So he invited his brothers and sisters in disease to join him on these hallway excursions. He believed that cancer patients, rather than languish all day atrophying, should get out of bed and move around. Thus, he went from room to room seeking recruits. Like him, many patients were undergoing chemo and radiation. Nevertheless, he found some takers. And on any given day, the Memorial staff could find Lebow ever the Pied Piper, leading a regiment of cancer patients speed-walking along his 200-yard hallway circuit, tile by tile.

After he left Memorial, he returned to the Central Park Reservoir for his runs. He was glad to get out among the curves and slopes of his beloved park, but he quickly realized that the cancer, the chemo, and the radiotherapy had slowed him down. "My pace dropped from about eight or nine minutes per mile to 15 or 16," Lebow recalled. "Between miles I would have to sit down for a minute or two. I would run in the park with a hood over my head so nobody would recognize me. I had no hair, no beard, and I had no interest in calling attention to my disease."

He was far from being in the clear. "I used to walk up the 10 floors to my apartment, even run up," he said. "Once, I made the trip in only 39 seconds. But sometimes, while getting chemo, I took the elevator up and went down by the steps. I became much weaker. I lacked the stamina I had before. I was afraid that if I climbed up, I might collapse between floors and nobody would find me."

"Sometimes," he said, "I would feel like staying in bed and sleeping rather than running. I would not even want to walk. But I felt it was healthier for me to go out. My body ached for motion. Every day my body was asking me to take it out, like a dog asking its owner to go out for a walk. From my home to Central Park is about half a mile, and sometimes I would start toward the park, feeling I should not do it. But I never turned around and went home. Never.

"At one point, I thought about how I might have only six months to live and had never run the five-borough marathon in New York City, and how much I wanted to. I'd run practically every other major marathon in the world: Chicago, Philadelphia, Los Angeles, Miami, Moscow, Paris, Rome, Helsinki, Seoul, and Stockholm. I'd run marathons in 35 countries. But never my own. One night, while taking my radiation and chemo, I felt I would never do it. And that made me feel bad."

❦ ❦ ❦

Through the 1980s, Lebow continued to bring to the job an obsession with detail that flirted with neurosis. Two weeks before each annual marathon, he would go out late at night, for several nights in a row, with a Department of Transportation crew. He would supervise the painting of the dotted blue line that the runners would follow along the streets and sidewalks. He would even lay down a few brush strokes on the pavement himself. On the day of the race, usually held in the morning on the first Sunday in November, he would ride in a convertible pace car, with all the marathoners following him, waving and shouting directions through a megaphone, by turns kindly and ruthless, always single-minded. "Fred is a perfectionist," his sister Sarah explained, "and that's what makes him very tough. He expects himself to do everything and to do it right, and the same goes for everyone else, too."

To administer the details of such an undertaking as the New York City Marathon quickly mushroomed into a task of unprecedented, if not daunting, complexity. In 1981, for example,

more than 100 buses were necessary simply to carry all the entrants
to the start of the race at the Verrazano Bridge in Staten Island.
The New York Road Runners Club needed to recruit 1,460 police
officers to monitor the procession of runners and had to shut
down 360 intersections throughout the city. So many runners
registered that the pistol for starting the race lacked the decibel
punch as a signal, so Lebow obtained from the U.S. Army a 75-
millimeter howitzer that emitted a blast approximating a sonic boom.

The New York City Marathon had caught on. In 1987 a
computer would spit out statistics underlying the marathon that
were astronomical: 41,900 applicants from all 50 states and 65
countries; 22,000 medals; 7,000 race-day volunteers, including
1,500 course marshals and 1,760 medical personnel; 440 portable
toilets; 4,000 roses; 18,000 yards of barricade tape; 20,000 feet of
rope; 33,110 T-shirts; 88,000 safety pins; 284 gallons of paint (for
the dotted blue line tracing the course); 30 medical units; 1,200
stretchers; 1,650 blankets; 582 tubes of K-Y Jelly; 22,000 cups of
coffee; 1.5 million paper cups for water or juice; 4 tons of ice; 2.5 tons
of bagels; and, of course, at least 37,000 Milky Way candy bars.

Today, the New York City Marathon remains the centerpiece
of the New York Road Runners Club. The winners of the event—
Alberto Salazar, Grete Waitz, Bill Rodgers, Rod Dixon, among
others—amount to a Hall of Fame for long-distance runners. The
marathon has grown to be an international event emulated by
cities everywhere. During the last 20 years, membership in the
club swelled from 270 to 28,000. With its $10 million annual
budget, the organization is the largest of its kind on the planet. It
stages more than 150 running events each year, including the
Fifth Avenue Mile and a dash up the Empire State Building, as
well as clinics and classes.

As a result, Fred Lebow is acknowledged as a pioneer in long-
distance running, his name synonymous with the modern
marathon. It is he, more than anyone else, who brought to bear a
genius for organization and a passion for running, that elevated
the ancient marathon to the status of 20th-century spectacle.
"When I organized the marathon in Central Park, I kept thinking,
It'll be a fly-by-night affair, it'll soon be over," he recalled. "But it kept
growing and growing. And now we have no more room to grow."

❦ ❦ ❦

Lebow, a lifelong bachelor, discovered early that his almost
pathological preoccupation with running was incompatible with
long-term romance. In 1973, for example, he lived with a young

woman who wanted him to marry her, or at least promise he would. But he kept putting off a commitment. Then she gave him an ultimatum: "Decide by the end of the year to marry me or we part company." Lebow agreed, never anticipating that his running schedule might interfere with her plans to domesticate him.

The year passed without a verdict—until December 31. Lebow and his lover were invited to a black-tie dinner party to ring in the new year. She looked forward to this glamorous soiree, knowing that she would finally hear whether the couple had a future together. Lebow flew in from a business trip, the night bitterly cold, gusts of rain and sleet buffeting the airplane on its approach to LaGuardia Airport. Moments before the plane touched down, Lebow happened to scan his running log. He had pledged to himself that he would run no fewer than 2,500 miles that year, about seven miles a day. Abruptly he realized, as he traced his fingers over the figures, that he had fallen short by 19 miles.

Determined to right this wrong, Lebow hurried from the airport to the apartment he shared with his girlfriend. He found her already dressed for the party, gorgeous in a new evening gown. The dinner party would start at 8 o'clock. But Lebow, instead of showering and taking out his tuxedo, slipped into a running outfit, sheepish about this last-minute change of plan. "Darling," he pleaded to his paramour, "just these last 19 miles." And out the door Lebow dashed, still an escape artist, heading over to Central Park in the slashing cold and sleet of a December night in New York City.

He cantered along through the park, hearing the siren song that beckoned him toward a 2,500-mile tally for the year. He covered the 19 miles as fast as possible. Then, just to make sure the deed was well and truly done, Lebow continued on for an extra mile or two.

He returned to the apartment at 10:00 p.m., abashed at his own audacity. His girlfriend averted her eyes and refused to speak with him, her fury at this breach of manners hanging in the air like a frost. Lebow showered quickly and put on his tuxedo. The couple arrived at the party too late for the dinner but early enough for drinks and dancing. As the clock tolled midnight, with all the revelers laughing and kissing and hugging, Lebow looked around the party for his girlfriend. She was gone.

Thus jilted, in a comeuppance perhaps well-deserved, if not long overdue, Lebow began the new year walking alone down a Manhattan street with the sleet hailing down on his shameful head. Hoping to reconcile with her, he arrived at her apartment and discovered his suitcase out in the hall, conveniently packed, with the front door double-locked, obviously to bar his entrance. On his luggage was a note from the woman now rebuffing him. "As she had warned me," Lebow recalled, "we were through. It was my fault, of course. It always is. I was always in running clothes. Maybe she would have liked to see me wearing something else occasionally. I was not attentive enough to her. I was always distracted by running."

"After this, whenever I met a girl I liked, I always said, 'You're wasting your time being with me. This will never turn into marriage.' I always let women know they had no future with me."

At the bottom of the note his former flame had placed a disheartening postscript. She had evidently taken the liberty of looking in his daily running log and adding up all the numbers. "Your actual mileage for the year," she wrote, going for the jugular in this final showdown, "was 2,531."

❦ ❦ ❦

Dr. DeAngelis, at Memorial, observed Lebow closely for the next six months, impressed with his commitment to treatment, conventional and otherwise, and his resolve to recover. "All along, Fred was going to do everything he could to fight the cancer," she said. "His approach was very positive. He had a very good outlook, but he was also very realistic and appropriately concerned. He was really concentrating on doing everything he could do to help himself get better. Fred was up and about, able to go to the office, take care of his business, and generally feel about as good as you could expect under the circumstances. He responded very briskly to the chemo and radiation. This kind of chemotherapy began only about six years ago. We know that combining chemotherapy with radiation substantially improves the prognosis. The tumor responds quickly to treatment and can disappear relatively rapidly. We monitored his progress with periodic CAT and MRI scans of the head. The problem is that this disease can come back, and the challenge is keeping the patient in remission. He handled the chemotherapy quite well, and the radiation, too, for that matter. But again, the issue is to make the tumor stay gone."

Thanks to swift, effective therapy, the tumor in his brain apparently disappeared, and in September 1990 Dr. DeAngelis pronounced his cancer in remission, ending all treatments. "The doctors originally thought my tumor was inoperable," Lebow recalled. "But the chemo and radiation reduced it completely."

Dr. DeAngelis attributed this turnaround, at least in part, to reliance on exercise as a companion to traditional therapy, and also to an intangible force of will. "When Fred got sick with this disease, he was in very good overall physical condition and had no other medical problems," she explained. "I have no question in my mind that his general good health worked in his favor, and that it enabled him to tolerate the treatments better and helped him to make a good recovery. We know that the better the condition patients are in before they have to deal with an illness like this, the better they do. In my mind, it's clear that his physical activity and fitness are related to his running and all his exercise and are certainly indirectly helpful in contributing to his overall general health.

"Fred also definitely has a mental resiliency. If you are a very resilient person, it enables you to deal with cancer that much more effectively. He's a very strong man emotionally, and I think that enabled him to deal with this from a realistic and positive perspective. He never got depressed during treatment and recovery. He was very patient about regaining his prior level of physical activity, yet he still demanded of himself that he go out and run virtually every day and do everything he could to get back to his previous condition. His focus in life was, appropriately, on resuming all of his prior activities, including his exercise routine. That's the message here: a cancer patient can get his life back.

"The attitude of the patient can be very important and helpful," the doctor said. "Sometimes a very bad attitude can work against a patient. But you should not credit success in treatment, or blame lack of success, on patient attitudes. It sort of implies that patients need the right attitude to get well, and without it, they do not get well. That's a dangerous idea. It can be very harmful to think that one failed to get better for lack of the right attitude. But as a general rule, yes, certain traits definitely help people deal with changes, because an illness like cancer usually wreaks havoc. It turns your whole world upside-down, and it stays upside-down for quite a while. To be an athlete takes a lot of discipline and determination and mental toughness. And Fred has those necessary qualities in abundance. He's really in a separate category, physically and mentally. That's why he's succeeded as a cancer patient."

❦ ❦ ❦

Two years after Dr. DeAngelis declared his tumor to be history, Lebow moved his narrow, angular frame slowly and haltingly around his office at the New York Road Runners Club, seeming frail and older than his 60 years. He took small steps, almost shuffling, then sat at his desk, surrounded by photos of him with Pope John Paul III and Presidents Reagan and Bush, plus memorabilia from trophies, plaques, and certificates to videocassettes, running books, and caricatures of himself.

Fresh from a run in the park, Lebow was dressed in—what else?—a lightweight running suit. Telephones trilled in the background: calls from would-be race sponsors, invitations to pose for running magazines and appear in out-of-town marathons, an offer from a book publisher to write his autobiography. With his freckled face and salt-and-pepper beard, Lebow leaned back in his chair, a few fugitive strands of hair flattened across his head, his eyes sad without being resigned, his voice now a whisper, at times impossible to hear. He rubbed his hand across his face and yawned, obviously tired, and apologized for doing so. As he nibbled on ruggelah from a kosher bakery around the corner, he talked about how cancer had changed his life.

"I never even thought about cancer before," Lebow said. "It's a dreadful disease. It makes you feel so helpless. Nobody is immune from it. And I did not want to be intimidated by the knowledge that I had it.

"I used to be obsessed with everything I did—smuggling diamonds, designing knockoffs, tennis, running. But now I realize I have certain limitations. I no longer play tennis for 14 straight hours or ski in the middle of the night. I think this disease helped me to find myself. It has brought me closer to my family and friends. I used to be tougher on my staff, tried to be a one-man business, control everything from A to Z, every little detail, because I thought I would do a better job, because I thought I cared more than anybody else, because I thought I knew the business better. I would work on everything—even the banners and balloons in a race. I was always around the office, always here. Now I've learned to delegate. I've realized that besides my job, I also have my family and friends and my girlfriend. All this helps keep me alive. I wake up in the morning and thank God that I'm still here."

Long-time friend Richard Traum detected a difference in Lebow immediately after his tumor faded. "Fred has publicly addressed the issue of doing good for others for the first time," he said, "and he's changed policies at the club to raise funds for charity. He's become mellower, more reflective, more interested in people."

Girlfriend Heather Dominic also noticed changes in him. "He's gotten calmer, and maybe the shock of the illness had something to do with that," she said. "Of course, the people who surround and support him have had a positive effect on him, too. He's

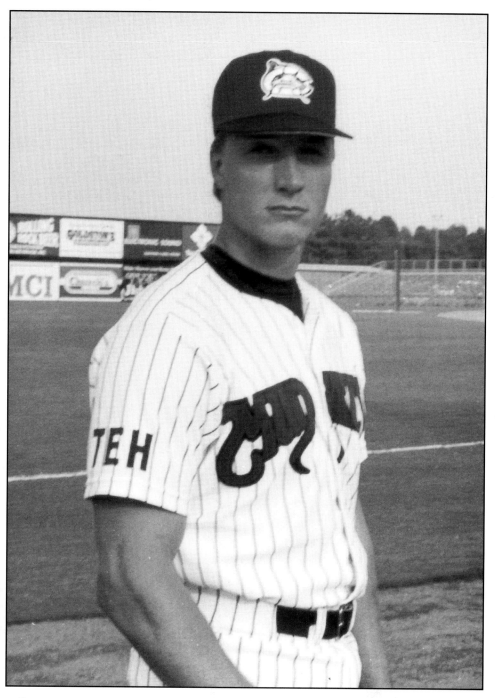

Jeff Banister played in the minor leagues for four-and-a-half seasons before the Pittsburgh Pirates beckoned. The tall Texan had survived seven surgeries for bone cancer on his left leg—and, a year later, a broken neck that left him paralyzed for ten days. "People have no idea how high a mountain I had to climb," he says. "I've received second and third chances, and for that I thank God."
Courtesy: Carolina Mudcats

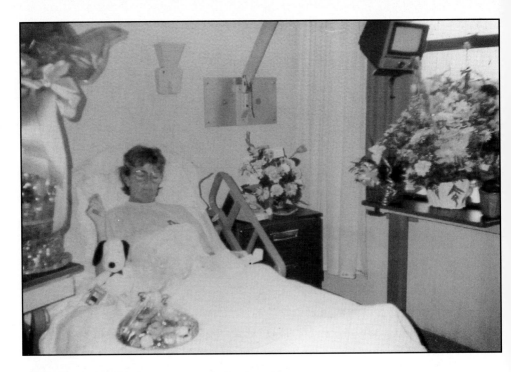

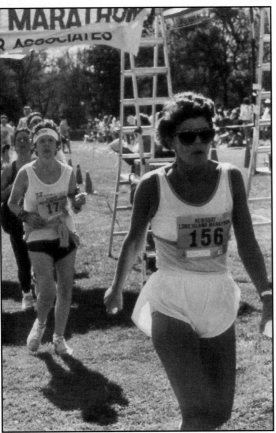

Long-distance runner Barbara Flores (above) was diagnosed with advanced ovarian cancer. "I constantly went up and down the halls at the hospital," she says. "That's all I ever did. I just wanted to get moving again."
Credit: Flores Collection

Flores (left) is still on the run today, competing mostly in 5K and 10K races and half-marathons. Here she completes Newsday Long Island Marathon, placing third in the 45–49 age group.
Credit: Flores Collection

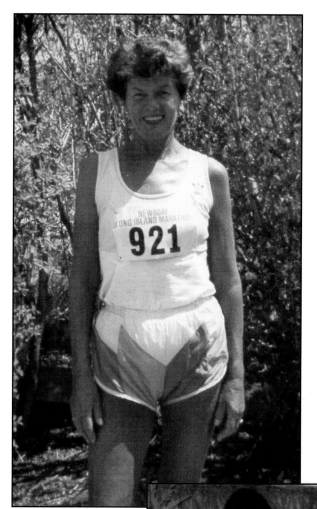

New Yorker Barbara Flores started running at age 41. Within a few years, she compiled a streak of victories in one-mile, five-mile, and half-marathon events.
Credit: Flores Collection

Barbara (below) toasting her close-call survival from cancer with husband, Ken, and children, Kevin and Cindy.
Credit: Flores Collection

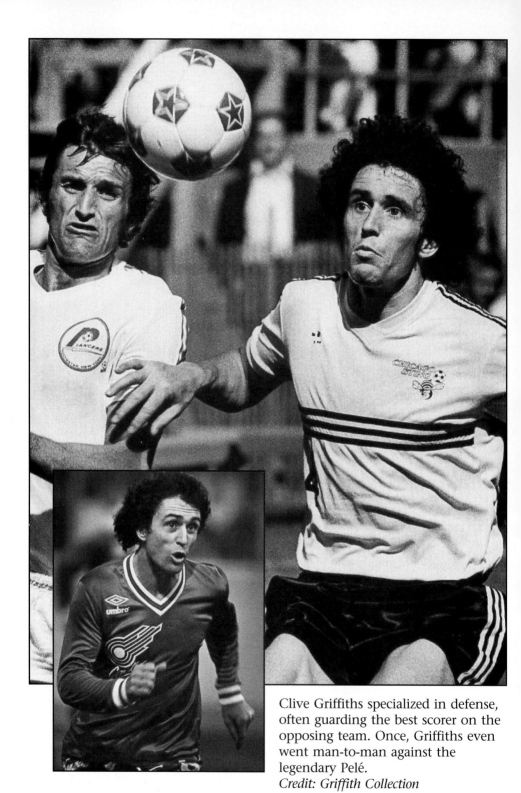

Clive Griffiths specialized in defense, often guarding the best scorer on the opposing team. Once, Griffiths even went man-to-man against the legendary Pelé.
Credit: Griffith Collection

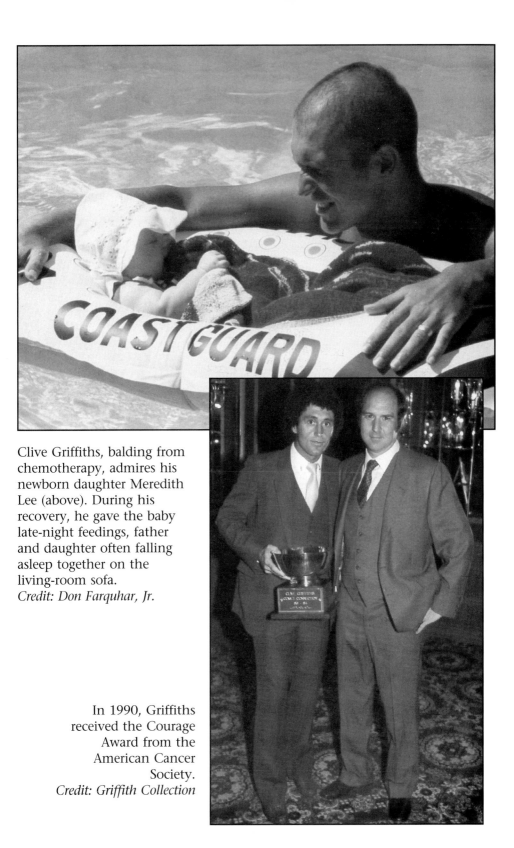

Clive Griffiths, balding from chemotherapy, admires his newborn daughter Meredith Lee (above). During his recovery, he gave the baby late-night feedings, father and daughter often falling asleep together on the living-room sofa.
Credit: Don Farquhar, Jr.

In 1990, Griffiths received the Courage Award from the American Cancer Society.
Credit: Griffith Collection

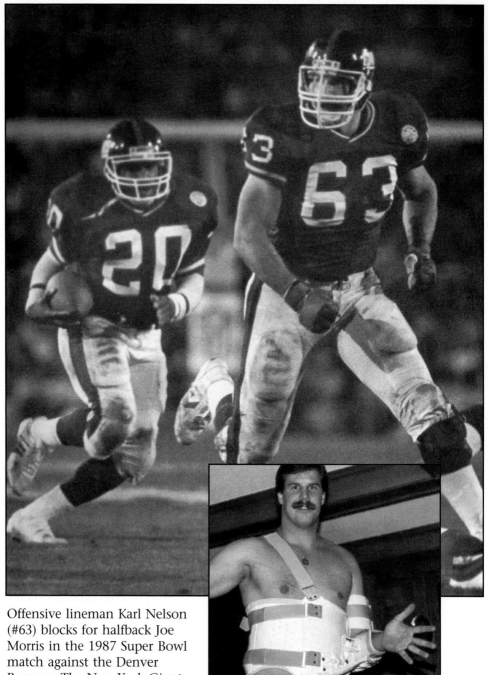

Offensive lineman Karl Nelson
(#63) blocks for halfback Joe
Morris in the 1987 Super Bowl
match against the Denver
Broncos. The New York Giants
scored on this march down field,
took the lead, and went on to
capture its first world championship in 30 years.
Credit: Jerry Pinkus
(below) Nelson wearing a brace after his shoulder surgery.
Credit: Nelson Collection

NFL standout Karl Nelson cuddles with his newborn daughter, Lyndsay, while recuperating from cancer. "All he wanted to talk about," says his wife, Heidi, "was how long it was going to take him to get back to playing football."
Credit: Nelson Collection

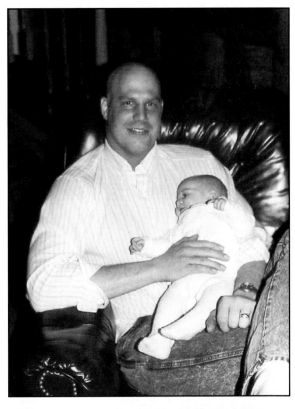

Nelson, now a radio sportscaster and financial advisor, shown here with wife, Heidi, and daughters, Brittany (left) and Lyndsay (right). He stays closely involved with Tomorrow's Children Fund, an organization that supports children who are afflicted with cancer.
Credit: Nelson Collection

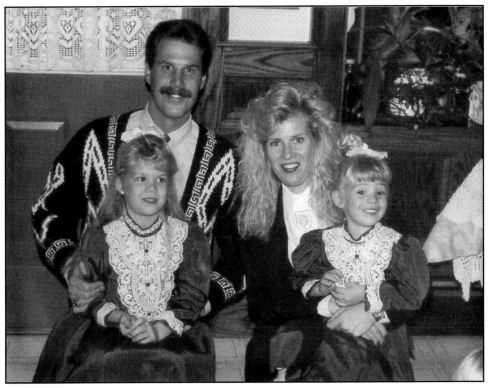

Fred Lebow (right), president of the New York Road Runners Club, built the New York City Marathon into the biggest, best-known event of its kind in the world. In 1992, the race had 25,945 contestants from 91 countries and 49 states. Fred is shown here with Dick Traum, his longtime friend and founder and president of the Achilles Track Club, an international organization for runners with disabilities.
Credit: Ken Levinson

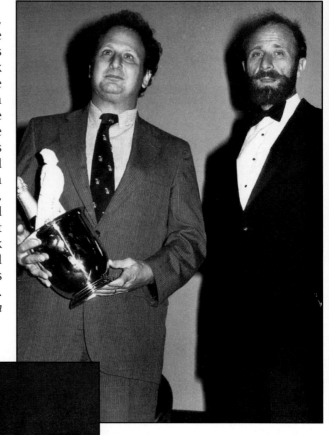

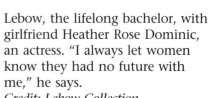

Lebow, the lifelong bachelor, with girlfriend Heather Rose Dominic, an actress. "I always let women know they had no future with me," he says.
Credit: Lebow Collection

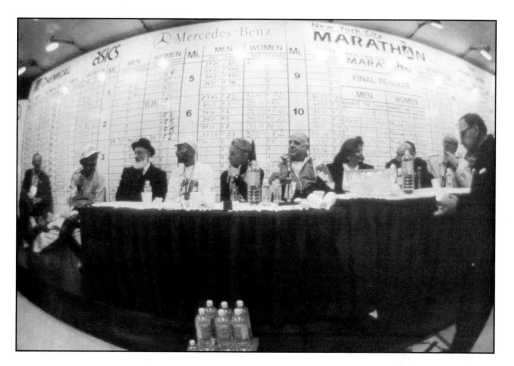

Lebow brought to the New York City Marathon an obsession with detail that flirted with neurosis. "Fred is a perfectionist," his sister Sarah explains, "and that's what makes him very tough." Two years after being told he would die within three to six months from an inoperable brain tumor, Lebow (right) completed the New York City Marathon. Grete Waitz, a close friend and nine-time female winner of the event, ran side-by-side with him in a gesture of support and affection.
Credit: Lebow Collection

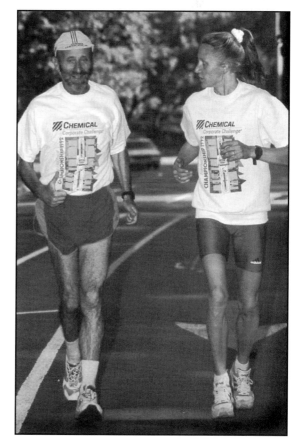

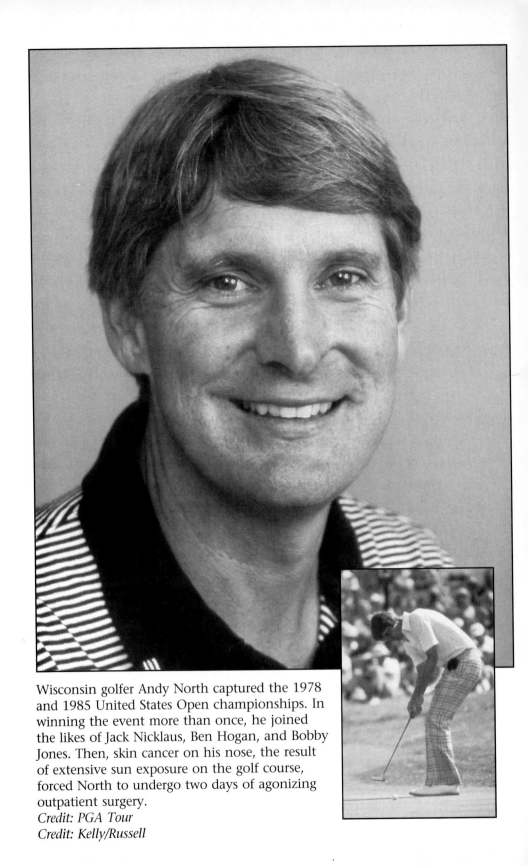

Wisconsin golfer Andy North captured the 1978 and 1985 United States Open championships. In winning the event more than once, he joined the likes of Jack Nicklaus, Ben Hogan, and Bobby Jones. Then, skin cancer on his nose, the result of extensive sun exposure on the golf course, forced North to undergo two days of agonizing outpatient surgery.
Credit: PGA Tour
Credit: Kelly/Russell

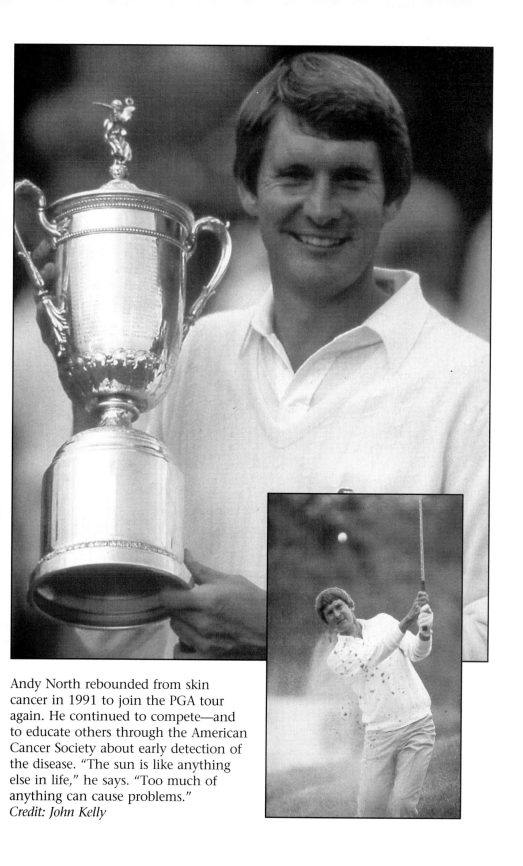

Andy North rebounded from skin cancer in 1991 to join the PGA tour again. He continued to compete—and to educate others through the American Cancer Society about early detection of the disease. "The sun is like anything else in life," he says. "Too much of anything can cause problems."
Credit: John Kelly

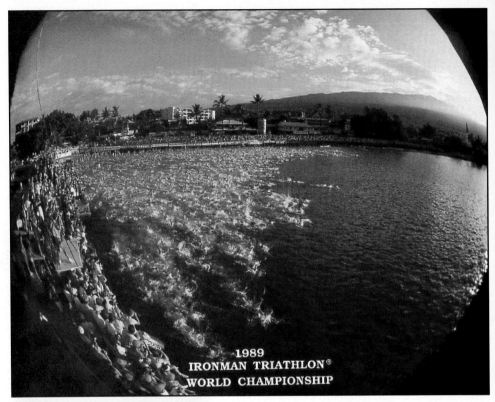

1989
IRONMAN TRIATHLON®
WORLD CHAMPIONSHIP

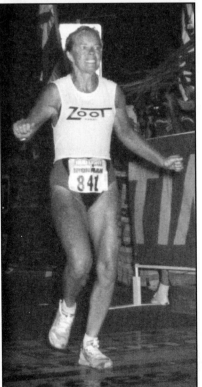

Connecticut attorney Barbara Norman, 51, completed the 1989 Bud Light Ironman Triathlon World Championship less than a year after treatment for breast cancer. She placed third in her age group in the event with a time of 13 hours, 14 minutes, 18 seconds. *Credit: Norman Collection*

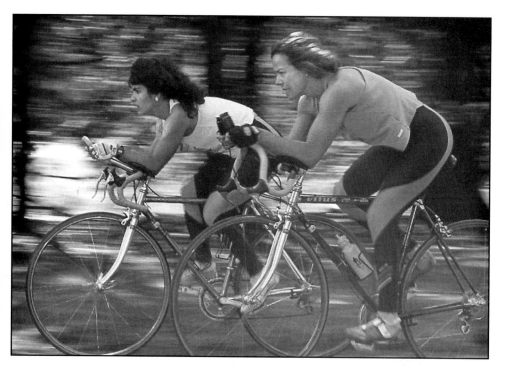

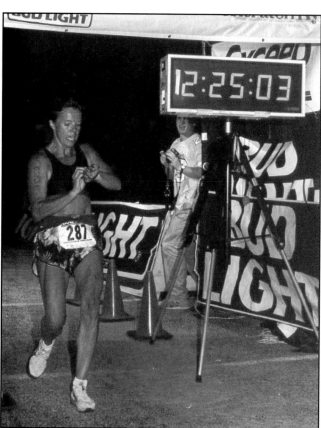

Barbara Norman (right, above) trained with friend and sister Kathy Bombace-Salvo, a stockbroker, 22 years her junior, while going through chemotherapy. "Kathy gave me a very special kind of support and encouraged me to compete," Barbara says. Norman (left) garnered first place in her age group at the 1988 Cape Cod Endurance Race, setting a new triathlon record for women 50–54 years of age. *Credit: Norman Collection*

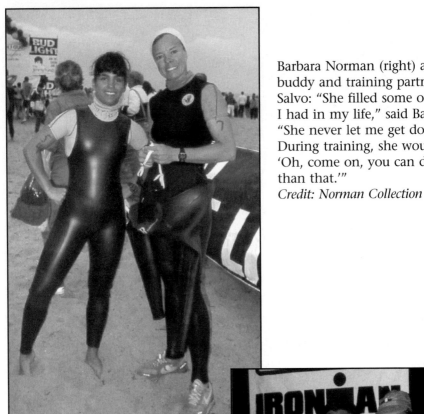

Barbara Norman (right) and buddy and training partner Kathy Salvo: "She filled some of the void I had in my life," said Barbara. "She never let me get down... During training, she would say, 'Oh, come on, you can do better than that.'"
Credit: Norman Collection

A triumphant Barbara Norman (center) shares her victory with family and friends.
Credit: Norman Collection

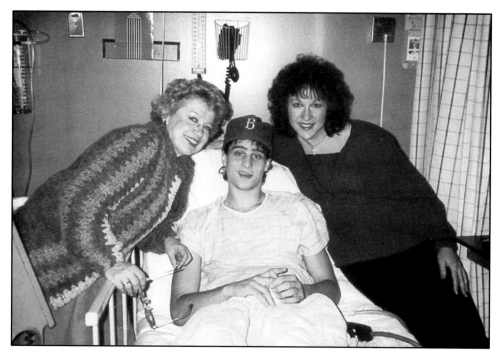

Handball champion Jason Vale, shown here with his mother, Barbara (left), survived a rare, often-fatal tumor and became a leading arm wrestler. *Credit: Vale Collection*

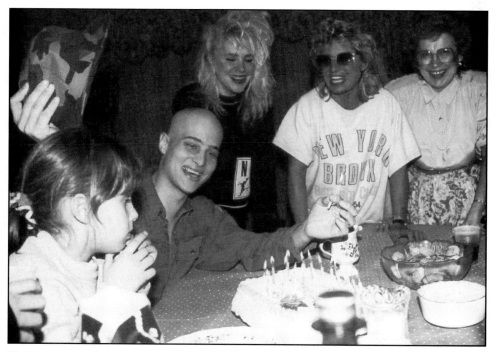

Vale, still sick from chemotherapy, celebrates his 19th birthday with family and friends. *Credit: Vale Collection*

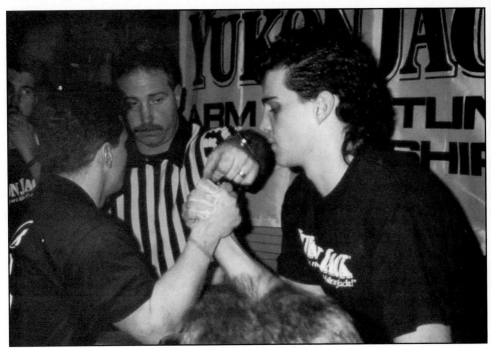

Jason Vale (right) is nicknamed Lightning Bolt because he pins arm-wrestling opponents so fast. His father, Joe, taught him the sport at the age of ten. *Credit: Vale Collection*

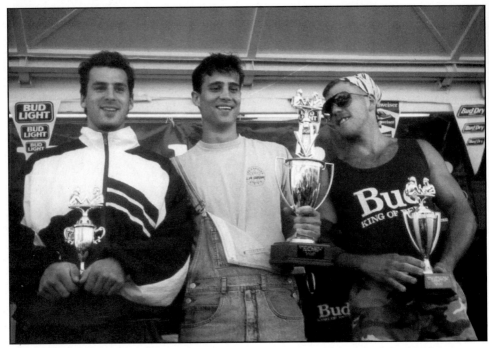

Vale won his weight division in the 1991 and 1992 Bud Light New York Pro Invitational Arm Wrestling Championship at the Queens Day Festival in New York City. *Credit: Vale Collection*

done a major turnaround with his family. Major. He's just gone straight ahead without letting the cancer interfere, without feeling sorry for himself. I've never seen him feel sorry for himself. He's managed the club, pushed programs, developed new plans and projects. He's gone through a life-threatening illness and still maintained everything else in his life and kept himself healthy.

"He's also become more open. He originally told me that when he found out about his illness, he never cried. But recently, he told me that when the doctors gave him the diagnosis, he did cry."

After his cancer treatments, Lebow also reverted, at least marginally, to the Judaism he had all but abandoned decades earlier. "Before, my attitude was: religion, who needs it?" he said. "I used to belittle it. I was brought up a very religious Jew. But I hated Hebrew school, hated it terribly, and I was a bad student. In the past, Jewish people would call to invite me to banquets and functions and usually I said no. Now I usually say yes. I feel a little more humble and spiritual now. I believe in God. I go to temple more often. I read more Jewish books. I'm definitely a stronger Jew than I was 10, 20 years ago. I feel more of a kinship now to other Jews. Respect for religion and its tradition have calmed me and made me more aware of the need for compassion toward others. It also makes me feel a bit more responsible for other people. I realize that I am not a man here by myself but that I exist within a world community of other people."

Cancer had partitioned Lebow's life. He had Life Before Cancer; now he had Life After Cancer. One is never the same. It's as if the disease had bled all arrogance from him, leaving a distillate of wisdom and understanding about priorities. For Lebow, survival of cancer—and its threat of finality—recast his life, streamlined it down to essentials. God. Brothers and sisters. An adoring girlfriend, whom he in turn adored. His job. Running. Still, even now, Lebow remained a hustler. Never taking no for an answer, he had negotiated with cancer. Cut a deal with death. "Why is Fred Lebow still here?" Brian Crawford said. "Because he wants to be."

❦ ❦ ❦

During recovery, Lebow took advantage of opportunities to reach out to other cancer patients. "Right after I left the hospital, people who were sick with cancer began to call me and write me letters," he said. "Or I would hear from a relative or friend of a patient; suddenly someone they loved was hit by cancer, and they needed a layman to explain what it meant. I've had a few hundred calls and letters. A father might call and say, 'I read about you, and I prayed for you, and I appreciate what you have done. My daughter is sick with cancer. Can you talk to her?'"

"You cannot hang up on these people," Lebow said. "At first I was dumbstruck that they called me. I think they see me as a successful cancer patient and think I'm an expert. They believe I can relay why I'm successful against cancer. But I say to patients, 'All I can really tell you about is my own experience. I cannot give you drugs or referrals to doctors, and I cannot give you miracles or say whether you should have a mastectomy. You have to understand that the doctors can do only so much. At some point you have to help yourself. Do some exercise to keep yourself physically fit and feel better mentally. And if you want to be healthy, you should also show that you want to be a part of this world. It's very important always to be engaged in something. Be busy. The only really happy people are busy people.'

"Knowing I can offer support and help people makes me feel better," Lebow said. "We have to force our limits in order to become stronger. By that I mean you keep pushing yourself even if you're half asleep or your legs are tired. You reach what you think is your limit and then you get a second wind and keep going. I want to try to get a message to other cancer patients: Look at me. I had cancer and I fought it. One time, a father called me about his 12-year-old son, who had cancer. The boy loved playing basketball with his father, but he had stopped because of his cancer. I spoke to the boy, and he sounded so sad that he could no longer play. He just felt too weak even for his shot to reach the basket. I said to him, 'How do you know you can no longer play? Just pick up the ball and bounce it a couple of times. No need to reach the rim. You could pretend to shoot at the hoop.' The boy listened, and a few weeks later his father called me. The boy had gone out to the basket in the driveway. For two weeks he dribbled and shot and tried to get the ball in the hoop. And finally he had. That's what his father wanted to tell me: that his son had tried again and again to reach the basket—until one day he got the ball in."

❦ ❦ ❦

Less than two years after he remembered the stolen chick, Fred Lebow decided to run in the 1992 New York City Marathon. It would be the first time he would compete in the event since it had fanned out to the five boroughs of the city. "My first year out of the hospital I could not have run the race—it was out of the question," he said. "But my second year, it seemed more possible."

Lebow began serious training—around the Central Park Reservoir, of course. As always, he would enter the park near the Metropolitan Museum of Art, head north around the reservoir, along the East Drive, up into Harlem, back down West Drive, past the reservoir again, toward the opulent Tavern on the Green restaurant, around a section known as the Dairy, and back toward headquarters. He shambled along either the two-mile or the four-mile loops. Even after all these years, his running style defied the laws of biomechanics. He still chugged along so erect he appeared to be starched, barely lifting his knees, pumping his arms too much.

For Lebow, the expansive greensward spread out like a welcome mat, with skyscrapers as its backdrop, almost like a set in a movie studio. He usually vied for passage along the running paths with the casual strollers, the race walkers, the bicyclists, the skate boarders, the roller bladers, and the high-speed baby buggies hauled along with a clickety-clack by fast-track mommies. Central Park continued to be a place where Fred Lebow, no less so than anyone else, went to lift his spirits.

"I think of Central Park as my back yard," Lebow said. "I probably know every nook and cranny of the six-mile course. I know all the people in the park. People come over to talk while I'm running. I listen, but I never want to talk while I'm running. So I say, gently, 'I cannot talk to you now. I'm running.'"

Every morning since leaving Memorial, Lebow grunted through a calisthenics routine of his own devising. The 10-minute warm-up program involved pushups and a maneuver that combined sit-ups with leg raises and light hand-held weights. "It's almost a religious ritual for Fred," Heather Dominic said. "Even when we travel—and his schedule is always crazy—he always sets aside time for his exercises. Fred really believes in his heart that the running and calisthenics keep him going. It really became a symbol of his commitment to get better—and stay well."

Slowly his appetite, dulled and all but destroyed by chemo and daily radiation treatments, returned full force. Lebow made a point of chowing down largely on fruit, vegetables, and pasta. Every morning, he sliced open two grapefruits and an orange and squeezed himself a glass of juice. On a typical day, he might put away a walnut-and-raspberry muffin for breakfast, a sandwich of Swiss cheese with lettuce and tomato for lunch, and a heaping bowl of pasta for dinner. To supplement the natural nutrients he took in, he daily popped A, B, and C vitamins. Given his furnace-like metabolism, he practically had to gorge himself to raise his weight five pounds to a still-thin 144.

Lebow resolved that the 1992 New York City Marathon would benefit Memorial Sloan-Kettering Cancer Center. In 1991 he had raised $652,173 for Memorial through the annual event. Now, in 1992, he and the renowned institution planned to generate more than $1 million through the run and mail-in donations. Lebow would be a designated runner, with donors pledging contributions based on the number of miles he completed. More than purely altruistic, this idea was a promotional masterstroke from the Barnum of road racing, certain to excite the sympathies of the city and arouse more interest in the race than ever before. The question was, could this fragile cancer survivor run a marathon?

"I think it's a definite possibility that Fred Lebow will run the New York City Marathon this year," Dr. DeAngelis of Memorial predicted. "I see nothing wrong with his striving to train to get back up to marathon level. I see no medical reason to stop him from trying it. On the contrary, he has every reason to believe he can."

"But a marathon is not a trivial undertaking. I'd be very cautious about saying this is what all cancer patients should do. Patients usually have to be very careful. If they are undergoing treatment such as heavy chemotherapy, they are usually not in a position to be able to exercise, and putting themselves through a lot of stress would be counterproductive. We have to be very cautious about blanket statements, because exercise for some patients should be encouraged, but for others it would be harmful. No patient with cancer, even if it's in remission, should undertake a vigorous exercise program without consulting a doctor."

Nobody questioned his decision. But a marathon, especially for a recovering cancer patient pushing 60 years old who had last run the distance four years earlier, was still a tall order, as Lebow quickly found out. "In training I have my ups and downs," he said. "But I'm a good patient. Each of us has to be smart when our body speaks to us and tells us something. Sometimes your body tells you to run five miles, other times only four miles."

"Cancer has changed my perspective," he said. "I still want to break seven minutes for a mile. I once ran seven-minute miles in a 10-kilometer race. But now my time is no longer important. I get more pleasure out of running now, even though I'm slower. Running is a gift, a treat I give to myself. Now if I break a 10-minute mile, I'm excited. I get more pleasure as a sick man running a 10-minute mile than I did as a healthy one running a seven-minute mile. Sometimes it hurts when I run. The first mile is always difficult, but then you get into a rhythm and start running like a locomotive. But the desire to run is so much stronger now. What's interesting is, you never lose that drive."

Brian Crawford believed his friend would pull off this act of faith. "It's his attitude," he said. "Fred thinks he can handle anything. Start a marathon in Central Park? Sure. Start a five-borough marathon? You bet. Beat cancer and run 26 miles? Hey, no problem."

Heather Dominic was convinced that if Lebow could come through brain cancer, surely he could go the distance in his 69th marathon. "I have no doubt that he's going to finish the marathon this November," she forecast. "It's something internal—something inside his body, his mind, his heart, his spirit—that keeps him running. That comes from what he went through as a child. He escaped from the Russians at the age of 13 and was separated from his family and traveled through Europe without any money. That's pretty intense. And that develops certain characteristics that stay with you. An instinct for survival, for relying on your own wits and strengths. He very much believes in self-determination. In running, you rely only on yourself and build an inner strength."

"Fred wants to run the five-borough marathon this year because he feels that right now is the time," Dominic said. "He's never done it and he wants to do it while he can. It's that simple. He keeps saying this may be his last marathon. But you never know."

❦ ❦ ❦

Lebow ground out three to six miles a day, about 30 per week, with some fifteen- and twenty-mile jobs on weekends, to boost his stamina as the big event approached. As tune-ups, Lebow ran a few 10-kilometer races and several half-marathons. In July 1992 he completed a 13.1-mile course in Siberia, of all places, and clocked a 2:17, about 10 minutes per mile; such a time translated, roughly, into a full marathon of about five hours, more than an hour slower than his personal best.

"After I ran six half-marathons, I realized I was ready for a full one," he said in early September 1992. "I think of myself as a one-man experiment. I dream about running the race, and it's scary. I visualize myself struggling about 15 or 18 miles into the race and hitting The Wall. I see myself wrapping my knees and ankles when they flare up. I see myself walking up all the hills. I cross the finish line and raise my hands. It may take me a long time to finish it this year, probably about five or six hours. I might even have to walk the last 10 miles. But I'll finish it. All I

want is never to come in last. And I think it will be my last
marathon. I want to carry a message to other cancer patients: Yes,
I had cancer. But now I'm in remission. And I can finish a
marathon."

※ ※ ※

On Sunday, November 1, 1992, at 10:48 a.m., with the
temperature a crisp 42 degrees and the sky an immaculate blue,
the cannon at Fort Wadsworth on Staten Island gave off a single
blast, and Fred Lebow, 32 months after cancer struck him,
embarked on his first five-borough New York City Marathon. He
wore Number 60, emblematic of his age, and ran side by side
with Grete Waitz, a close friend and nine-time female winner of
the event, who, in a gesture of sentiment, accompanied Lebow
on the understanding that she would move at about half her
usual pace. "I saw Fred two years ago," the Norwegian champion
said. "He looked so sick, and I felt so sorry for him. I heard he
had only six months to live. I never thought that two years later
he would be running a marathon."

Lebow tottered along, also accompanied by 25,945 other
entrants, runners from 91 countries and 49 states. He and Waitz
were immediately surrounded by course marshals, friends, and
members of the media, who clustered around him in an entourage
intended to serve as a protective membrane. Nobody wanted an
overenthusiastic fan to sidetrack this famous recovering cancer
patient. "It's my job to tell spectators to leave him alone," Waitz
said.

Among the estimated two million spectators lining the race
course were his brothers Shlomo, Michael, Morris, Simcha, and,
of course, his devoted sister Sarah. It was the first time his family
had gathered expressly to see him run. Lebow had come prepared
to concentrate on the race, even to the extent of wearing earplugs.
He had also rehearsed a thumbs-up signal with both hands, to
acknowledge the cheers he anticipated and spare him the energy
of waving to crowds of well-wishers.

WABC-TV would broadcast the event for the next four-and-a-
half hours, with the WCBS radio station carrying continuous
coverage and others giving frequent updates. All along the route,
from the Verrazano Bridge to Central Park—indeed, throughout
New York City—citizens waited for word, all the fans and race
volunteers and city workers united by a single overriding interest.
"Where's Fred?" everyone wanted to know. "How's he doing?"

Lebow was doing okay. A thin, bewhiskered figure in a lime-yellow bicycle racing cap and neon blue running suit with long pants, he cruised across the Verrazano Narrows Bridge, from Staten Island into Brooklyn, and tottered along Fourth Avenue for the first five miles past Prospect Park. The first few miles came easy for him. Brooklynites looking on cheered him, the earplugs he wore somewhat muting the chorus, and Lebow gave his much-practiced thumbs-up sign.

As he approached Williamsburg, a community largely made up of orthodox Jews, even today reminiscent, with its tiny shuls and cloaked Talmudic scholars, of a 19th-century Eastern European village before the Diaspora. Lebow felt a twinge of kinship. The Hasidic Jews along the route shouted out "shalom" to him, and he returned the greeting in kind. It warmed him to be urged on by standard-bearers for the Judaism he had lost in his flight from Nazis and Communists, only to find his religion all over again when near death.

Lebow plodded on for five more miles along Lafayette and Bedford and Manhattan Avenues in Brooklyn, his mode of locomotion still awkward, his feet barely rising off the pavement, his arms cranking stiffly. Spectators rubbernecked to catch a glimpse of him and screamed his name. Race volunteers rushed out to him holding cups of soup, orange slices, and candy bars. Someone held a sign saying LEBOW FOR PRESIDENT.

At about 1:00 p.m., Lebow crossed the Pulaski Bridge, the halfway point for the race, and headed into Queens. By now, South African Willie Mtolo had won the event in 2:09:29, and a few minutes later Australian Lisa Ondieki hit the tape in 2:24:40. Each winner collected $20,000 in prize money and a Mercedes.

Lebow was no longer the same runner as before. He ran slowly, he ran with difficulty, but at least he ran. He walked up the steep inclines leading to each bridge he crossed. After 13 miles, he was still in the race, the race of his life, weaker in body but stronger in spirit.

He trundled along Vernon Boulevard, then across the Queensboro Bridge into Manhattan. With 11 miles still left, he headed north along First Avenue to 138th Street, across the Willis Avenue Bridge into the Bronx. Only six miles left now. The race had a festive air about it, with no fewer than 25 bands playing along the course. One runner dressed as a rhinoceros to dramatize the plight of that endangered species. But some spectators dashed onto the course in attempts, ultimately aborted, to shake hands with Lebow or run in formation with his retinue. One interloper tried to stop Lebow long enough to pose for a photo.

After 21 miles, the chronic pain in his knee flared up, and Lebow strapped on a brace. He went over the Madison Avenue Bridge and back, down to Fifth Avenue, and around Marcus Garvey Park. The escape artist stopped running about every two miles to walk. Then he turned off Fifth Avenue at 102nd Street and entered Central Park, signaling the homestretch. Passing Memorial Sloan-Kettering Cancer Center, he waved to the hospital staff and looked among the faces, without luck, for Dr. Lisa DeAngelis. Waitz sensed that around this point Lebow began to beam, as if he sniffed the finish line. As Norwegians put it, Waitz later said, *Gamle sirkushester lukter sagmugg.* Translation: old circus horses smell the sawdust.

Even now, hours after the front-runners had finished, the crowd lining the course in Central Park remained thick. Now the Lebow entourage was spearheaded by police cars, support vehicles, and TV camera operators. Lebow toddled along elegant Central Park South and cut back into the park. As he approached the finish line, near West 67th Street, spectators gathered to watch him come full circle. The finish line was, in a sense, where it had all begun for him nearly 20 years earlier.

New York City Mayor David M. Dinkins held the finish-line tape at one end, male winner Willie Mtolo at the other. Lebow snapped the tape under a canopy of golden leaves, arm in arm with Waitz, and received the longest, loudest cheer of the day. He finished with a time of 5:32:34, almost exactly between the five and six hours he had predicted. And now he and Waitz kissed each other and cried. Mayor Dinkins greeted and hugged him. Lebow dropped to his knees and kissed the finish line.

In 490 B.C., more than two millennia ago, an Athenian runner named Pheidippides had carried out a mission that left an indelible mark on the history of sports. The city of Marathon had dispatched him to Athens with the news that the Persian army had suffered a terrible defeat. The original marathon man had covered the 25 miles from the battlefield to the capital at top speed, delivered his message, and dropped dead. Unfortunately, in running this distance, Pheidippides had found death. Lebow, on the other hand, had found life. And in so doing, he, too, had delivered a message.

Chapter 6

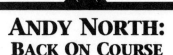

ANDY NORTH:
BACK ON COURSE

Here comes the sun, hot as hell, its surface sizzling at 10,000 degrees Fahrenheit, more than 20 times the heat needed to grill a steak. This star shimmers with the light and heat that support life on earth, an immense globe of luminous gas, more than 4.6 billion years old, synonymous with growth and replenishment. From sunlight originates our very climate, much of our fuel, and some of our food. Doses of sun ward off depression and lethargy, relieve psoriasis, acne, and aching joints, and better enable our bodies to metabolize Vitamin D.

But for all the good it does, the sun spells bad news for human skin. The skin is the largest organ of the body, covering about 20 square feet on the average adult human. A thin sheaf, between one-fourth and one-thirty-second of an inch thick, the skin is fraught with nerve endings, hair follicles, sweat glands, and cells. Its job is to protect other organs, retain moisture, and, most of all, to protect against infection, harmful chemicals, and, yes, radiation.

The sun, of course, emits radiation, beaming down ultraviolet light (UV), invisible rays in the light spectrum that are radioactive. Overexposure can not only make skin lose its elasticity but also leave it hard, thin, and dry, with a wrinkly texture. Sunlight can also cause liver spots, dark patches called actinic keratosis, and that most dreaded disease—skin cancer. The sun triggers at least 90 percent of all cases. Here comes the sun, and there goes the skin.

Andy North knows firsthand what the sun can do. North plays golf for a living and, as such, is among the least likely inhabitants of the planet to elude the sun. Golf is a sport played outdoors, in locales like California and Florida and Hawaii, places seldom eclipsed by shade. To play a round of golf, all 18 holes, typically takes about four hours, and a tournament calls for four such rounds. With most pro golfers competing in about 30 tournaments a year, they're in the sun about 10 hours a week (discounting preliminary rounds and practice time), often during midday, when the sun glares most fiercely.

Andy North has played on the Professional Golf Association tour for nearly 20 years, all 6 feet, 4 inches and 200 pounds of him, a good-looking Wisconsin boy now graying at 43. He's made quite a name for himself, too, capturing titles in two of the biggest golf tournaments around. But during all that time, during all those holes of golf, all those rounds in all those tournaments around the world, the sun baked him. He took precautions, but not enough, not nearly enough, and the sun scorched him. He never realized what the sun could do to his skin until it was too late and he had skin cancer.

As cancers go, no doubt it could've been worse, much worse. He would get through the disease without tubes coming out of his chest, without chemotherapy, without a stay in the hospital. His life was never threatened and his story contains no heroism, no miracles; it's mainly a story of the sun and the skin. What happened to him can happen to anyone, and it often does.

❦ ❦ ❦

As a little boy, Andrew Stewart North left the house early in the morning on Saturdays and Sundays and came home in the evening. In between, he played. Outdoors. All day. And every weekday after school, he played. That was what a kid was supposed to do; it was his job. He played baseball and basketball and football, played without ever seeming to get tired or hurt, played with the certainty that his body would always snap back. It was the 1950s and everyone loved the sun. "We never gave the idea of being out in the sun a second thought," he recalled. "You never thought about sunscreen because it was before they had any. It was the sun. How could it be bad for you? All of us kids, we just got barbecued."

As a rule, young children possess delicate skin, highly vulnerable to the damaging ultraviolet rays that cause most skin cancer. Most of the sun exposure that leads to skin cancer occurs during childhood. A Harvard study estimated that the average child in the United States gets three times more annual ultraviolet light exposure than the average adult. The process by which this exposure develops into skin cancer is insidiously cumulative and usually takes 20 to 30 years to manifest itself. Damage done in childhood may not show up until age 50—or, as in the case of Andy North, 41.

North encountered physical hardship early. When he was 12

years old, a bone in his right knee stopped growing and began to disintegrate. The family doctor diagnosed a bone disorder called osteochondritis dissecans, an inflammation in which a fragment of cartilage and its underlying bone become detached. He might have had to give up all sports—except his doctor found a loophole in this contract. Let's go down a list of sports, he told the boy, to determine which, if any, you can play. Okay, the seventh grader said. And the answer for a kid unable to walk was, of course, golf. All he could do was play golf, provided he rode around the course in a cart. That's how he started playing the sport: from a cart.

Luckily, his father, Stewart, could play golf—in those days, he boasted a handicap of three or four—and taught him the game. All through seventh and eighth grade, all through those 18 months that Andy hopped around everywhere he went on crutches, his father took him out on the links after work to ride around in a cart and play nine holes. His father showed him how to drive, how to chip, how to putt. Andy learned to align his body and send the dimpled ball—thwack!—flying toward the cup. He went out on his own, practicing late at night under the lights, pretending, in his frequent fantasies, that he was putting on the 18th green for first place in the U.S. Open.

As the boy improved, he came to like the game. "It was just you against yourself, you against the ball, you against the golf course, you against the elements," he said. And he kept at it, even after he resumed playing other sports. As a high school senior, he returned to basketball and earned all-state honors. But most of all he liked golf, the quietude of the fairways, the beauty of the freshly-cut greens, the challenge of self-control, the solitary peace of it all. "You have to enjoy spending time by yourself," he said. "Self-discipline is important. You're out there working on your game without anyone else around."

Shy and soft-spoken, North quickly proved that he could golf with the best. While a student at the University of Florida, he won the 1969 Wisconsin State Amateur and the 1971 Western Amateur, and for three consecutive years he ranked as a collegiate all-American. In 1972, he turned professional, and every year thereafter he improved. He won the 1977 American Express-Westchester Classic, garnering his first major tournament victory and a $60,000 paycheck. The next year, at the age of 28, he would break through to the upper echelon of pro golfers.

It happened at the 1978 United States Open Championship at Cherry Hills in Denver, where North assumed the lead early in the week. Going into the round on Saturday, he had a two-stroke advantage over none other than Jack Nicklaus. The next day, a guy named Gary Player tailgated North, two strokes behind. On the 13th hole of the final round, North sank a 15-foot putt and, with only five holes to play, he bolted ahead by five strokes.

Then he collided with his own worst enemy: himself. He bogeyed the 14th. He double-bogeyed the par-three 15th. Still leading on the 18th, he needed merely a bogey to win, but his tee shot caught the edge of the bunker, and it looked as if he might not even manage a bogey. Then he came through with what, to that point, was the biggest shot of his life. He chipped from the sand trap to within four feet of the cup, then putted in for a par. In winning this major tournament, North edged out Dave Stockton and J.C. Snead, no slouches, and collected a first prize of $45,000, not bad for a week at the office. "Ever since I was a kid, it was one of my goals to win the U.S. Open," North recalled. "But I also felt I was supposed to do it, that every year I would follow a natural progression and improve and earn more money. And that's what happened." He ended the year with $150,000 in winnings and 14th in the world.

Around this time, the sun flickered its first warning for Andy North. His father, who had grown up on a farm and spent most of his time outdoors in the Wisconsin sun, developed skin cancer. Leathery Stewart North noticed a spot on his face, went in to see his dermatologist and received treatment. Over the years he became a regular customer, needing minor—and not-so-minor—surgeries for the removal of pieces of himself, chunks of skin from his ears, nose, and arms.

Uh oh, Andy thought. Better watch out. And Andy, who, like his father, had pale skin, started putting on sunscreen before every golf outing. He slathered protective cream on his arms and face, especially on the protrusions of his lips, nose, and ears, and started wearing a cap, too, the better to save his skin. "Because of my father, I became so much more aware of skin cancer and stayed on top of it," Andy said. "His cancer made me want to take better care of myself."

North turned out to be an early proponent of ritual protective measures against the radioactive punishment of the sun. In 1978, the U.S. Food and Drug Administration first recommended labeling all sun-care products with a "Sun Protection Factor" or "SPF," a numerical code that indicates how much a product will protect you from the sun. The higher the SPF number, the more the product shields skin against UV rays and the longer one can sunbathe safely. A product designated with an SPF of six, for example, enables a person ordinarily likely to turn red after an hour of exposure to the sun to safely sunbathe for six hours, or six times longer than an hour, without burning the skin. Over the years, North has vigilantly applied an SPF 15.

In the late 1970s, North also became a volunteer for the Wisconsin chapter of the American Cancer Society. He raised funds, visited cancer patients, acted as a spokesperson, and promoted golf events, his mission to raise awareness of skin cancer and help educate the public. Little did he realize that in early middle age, he would develop the disease.

In the fall of 1983, pain in his right elbow—a crucial piece of equipment for a golfer—forced North to undergo an operation to remove a bone spur the size of a nugget of gravel, and over the next year he struggled on the tour, missing some tournaments. By 1985, seven years had passed since his victory at Cherry Hills, his only tour victory. Some observers were ready to write off North, only 35 years old, as a fluke, a one-tournament wonder.

But at the 1985 U.S. Open at Oakland Hills in Birmingham, Michigan, North again staked his claim as a golfer to be reckoned with. After the second round, he trailed the leader by three strokes; after the third, by only two. In the final round, on a cold, windy day, he was locked in a tight contest with Tze-Chung Chen, Dave Barr, and Denis Watson. On the 17th hole, North burst into the lead and went on to win the tournament by a single stroke, with a one-under-par 279. He received a $103,000 prize and erased the seven-year itch. In winning his second U.S. Open, North joined the elite company of Lee Trevino, Ben Hogan, Jack Nicklaus, Hale Irwin, Bobby Jones, and Gene Sarazen, the pantheon of legendary golfers who, since the tournament was first staged in 1903, had triumphed in the event more than once. North concluded 1985 with six top-10 finishes, earning $212,000 and ranking 24th in the world.

North has never walloped tee shots as far as, say, Greg Norman, never chipped out of sand traps as deftly as Ben Crenshaw, never putted as precisely as Watson or Nicklaus. Like many pro golfers, he could do it all pretty well. But more valuable than the right stroke, the strength in his wrists, eyesight almost radarlike in its acuity—more than his pure physical prowess, of which he undeniably had an abundance—Andy North was equipped with cool. He had a disposition custom-made for golf, because golf is a game that calls, above all else, for cool. It is a game of the utmost control and delicacy and exactitude. A sport for adults, really, it took maturity, almost a judicial demeanor. On a putt, a half an ounce too much pressure applied to the putter's handle will send the ball skittering an inch past the cup. Such an errant shot could cost tens of thousands of dollars in prize money. All from an extra half-ounce of pressure.

The key in golf is to stabilize the degree to which one becomes aroused. A theory called the Yerkson-Dodson Law dictates that the more complex the athletic task, the less psyched one should become. According to this idea, conceived by sports psychologists, complicated tasks are performed better when emotional drive is low, and vice-versa. To wit, intense drive is conducive to producing the explosion of strength needed in football, basketball and baseball, but one can excel at golf—or, for that matter, archery or billiards—only if one is tranquil enough to maintain precision, finesse, and a feathery touch.

Out on the links, North was among the coolest of the cool. The expression on his face never revealed whether his shot had gone arrow-straight or hooked or sliced. If he smiled on the golf course at all—and it was an infrequent occurrence—he smiled thinly and briefly. He spoke a language of neutrality and understatement, a dialect indigenous to pro golfers. If the day was going well, he tried not to soar too high; if it was going poorly, he tried not to sink too low.

North strode down the fairway, eyes fixed ahead, thinking only about the next shot, even as the gallery flocked around him, the TV cameras whirring, the commentators whispering to millions of viewers at home. North knew if you kept cool, you could hang in there, stay in the running for the big money, even on those inevitable days when your stroke was off half an ounce. You kept on an even keel. No foot-stomping, fist-pounding, hell-raising temper tantrums for Andy North. Cool. The sun got hot, but Andy North kept cool. Mr. Cool, through and through.

What tested that cool in golf more than anything else was not the shots themselves but, rather, the time between shots. There was so much time, so much time to think—no opportunity to rely on reflex, no spontaneity at all, everything calculated, deliberate, premeditated—and all that thinking could distract and disturb a golfer. "In baseball, you never have time to think about hitting a pitch or catching a line drive," North said. "Golf is one of the few sports where you never need to react to something somebody else is doing to you. We have too much time to think about what we're doing. If you over-evaluate, a lot of times you really get in your own way."

Soon North would have plenty of time to think about

something other than golf. For about three years now, he had needed to visit a dermatologist about once every six months. The doctor would find a slight abnormality on his face, a flat little freckle, like a liver spot, evidently nothing of long-term consequence, and either freeze or dissolve it with liquid nitrate, and that would be that, at least until the next visit. All those treatments offered a preview of the problem to come, but North never suspected the spots would get worse. He had taken precautions, smeared on the SPF 15, worn a cap, but it was too late.

All those days playing outside, days without end, and now the sun had gotten under his skin. Here came the sun, and there went his skin. Mr. Cool never expected to pay for taking too much heat.

❦ ❦ ❦

Susan, his wife of 19 years, noticed it first. In March 1991, at the Honda Classic in Coral Springs, Florida, the Norths were eating dinner. He was playing well, had regained his stroke, his rhythm, and was putting the package back together, finally, after a few consecutive years of difficulties. He had just come off a strong season in 1990, ranking higher than he had since 1985. By now, the game he had taken up as a 12-year-old, by default, had earned him more than $1.3 million.

Susan looked across the table at Andy and noticed that the left side of his nose seemed... well, different. Not a spot or a mole or lump or a nodule. Just something. Maybe its size. Maybe its shape. As the Norths progressed through the main course, Susan looked again, just to be sure. Is his nose different, she thought, or do I need bifocals? In the background, other diners murmured amid the clink and clatter of the meal. Should she say something to Andy or keep this perception to herself? It seemed so silly. How could his nose possibly be different? This was Andy North, not Michael Jackson. Better tell him, she thought.

"Your nose looks different," Susan said. "Something looks really wrong with it." This was a first, both for her to say it and for him to hear it.

"No," Andy said.

"Yes, I think so."

"Come on."

"Really. Your nose looks a little thinner."

"You're crazy. It's nothing."

"I want to call a doctor."

"Forget it."

"You could just let him take a look. Just go talk to him."

Back and forth they went, she contending, he denying. But Susan North could be as stubborn as he. They had started dating as seniors in high school, and he knew that. And after she took a plane home to Wisconsin, she had the initiative and foresight to make an appointment for her husband with Dr. Stephen Snow, a skin cancer specialist and associate professor of surgery at the University of Wisconsin Hospital in Madison. "I'd never done anything like that," she said. "I just felt certain that this time he should see a cancer specialist, not a dermatologist."

Andy returned home from the tournament a few days later and went in to see Dr. Snow, who examined his nose and left cheek and conducted two biopsies. The report from a pathologist revealed a lesion, flat, slightly wider in diameter than a dime and about half an inch deep, located in what is called the ala, the wing of the nose, along the groove just over the bump of his left nostril. Dr. Snow told North he had skin cancer—specifically, an advanced case of basal cell carcinoma, the most common, and least serious, of skin cancers. Like father, like son.

"We've found a problem," Snow told North, "and we need to work on it. We need to take this out. I want to get you back in here right away. You have a skin cancer. It's not the big 'C.' It will stay local. It will not spread to your internal organs. But if left untreated, it will invade underlying tissue on your face."

The physician knew North had to leave soon for another golf tournament and explained that he would need outpatient surgery. But he also assured the golfer that the lesion was probably no worse than the spots the dermatologist had found on his face over the years. Snow wanted to put North at ease, although he remained unsure of exactly what he might find during surgery.

Okay, North thought. It all sounded pretty casual to him, less than grave, so he hardly gave it a second thought. "When you hear the word cancer," Susan North said, "it's devastating, even if it's skin cancer, because we all know someone who died from cancer. Your life changes. But Andy had a so-what attitude. He figured, Oh, it's cancer, but at least we know. Like, Yeah, it's bad, but I'll go in as an outpatient and the doctor'll take care of it and just cut it out."

"I thought everything was going to be okay," North recalled. Every time the dermatologist had found a nagging little spot on his face over the last three years, he had zapped it off. That's how North phrased it: the doc zapped my spot. How bad could this business be? It was just outpatient stuff. No need for a CAT scan or chemo shots. Sure, it was cancer, North thought as he headed down to Jacksonville, Florida, for the Tournament Players Championship. But it was only *skin* cancer.

❦ ❦ ❦

Skin cancer is the most widespread, most easily preventable and, if detected early, most curable of all cancers. The condition afflicts more than 600,000 people in the United States every year, nearly half of all cancer cases recorded. Treated early, a vast majority of skin cancers—close to 95 percent—can be removed and cured. About 60 percent of cases involve basal-cell carcinoma, and 20 percent are squamous-cell growths. The rest are malignant melanomas, the most serious and least common, with about 5,800 cases that annually result in death. The incidence of melanoma has risen from one in 1,500 people in 1930 to one in less than 150 today, according to the Skin Cancer Foundation, and will increase to one in 100 by the year 2000.

What provokes skin cancer? In response to UV rays, tiny granules of melanin, a brownish pigment made in specialized skin cells, rise to the surface and try to act as sunlight deflectors. But after prolonged exposure, the UV rays cause the basal cells near the surface of the skin to swell and the blood vessels to dilate and turn red. Long-term buildup of melanin in the skin's underlying layers damages cells that produce the collagen, which gives skin its resilience and structure, and elastin fibers, which create its pliability.

People with fair skin, light hair, and blue, green or gray eyes—the Irish are an obvious example—face a higher risk than others. Farmers, sailors, fishermen, construction workers, and others who work under the sun are also more vulnerable to carcinomas. Black people rarely suffer from the disease. More men than women get it, probably because more men work outdoors. The closer one lives to the equator, the higher the likelihood of skin cancer. Also, because of its long-term, cumulative effects, more old than young people contract the disease.

About 90 percent of all skin cancers occur on sites of the body left exposed, usually the face, the lips, the tips of the nose and ears, the hands, and the forearms. But in the last 50 years or so, as more people have sunbathed and received higher doses of sunlight, more skin cancers have shown up on the shoulders, backs, and chests of men and the lower legs of women. Treatments include freezing, electrical currents, radiation therapy, and surgery.

Basal-cell carcinoma, the version that struck North, is typically found in the middle-aged and elderly, the result of extensive, prolonged exposure to the sun. Slow-growing, it usually appears as a small, shiny, pearly bump or nodule on the head, neck, or hand. If left untreated, the tumor can bleed and crust over, only to pop open again. Rarely does it spread and threaten life, but it can reach and destroy underlying tissue. The deeper under the skin it penetrates, the more likely it is to metastasize. Such tumors can migrate to the lymph glands and organs such as the lungs, bone and brain. A tumor undetected and untreated for too long can mean scarring or disfigurement, including the loss of an eye, an ear or a nose.

Only skin cancer?

❧ ❧ ❧

On March 22, back from the tournament in Florida, North appeared for his appointment with Dr. Snow at the University of Wisconsin Hospital. The golfer would need what is called Mohs' surgery. Named after inventor Frederick Mohs, the procedure is frequently performed on recurring growths or tumors on locations that are difficult to reach by other surgical means, such as the eyelids, the nose, or the helix of the ear or lips. In a Mohs procedure, the surgeon slices away the skin one thin sliver at a time, in a circle about one-sixteenth of an inch thick, to remove the tumor. Then each layer is turned upside-down and scanned under a microscope. And so on, layer by layer, similar to peeling an onion, until the growth is gone. The idea is take out no more nor less than necessary, preserving normal, healthy tissue while removing the cancerous sections, thereby sharply lowering the risk of spread or recurrence.

North reclined in a body-length padded chair with armrests, like the kind you see on a visit to the dentist. Dr. Snow hovered over him and inserted a hypodermic needle into the left side of his nose, slowly pressing the cylinder of the syringe to inject North with anesthetic to numb that region of his face. Then he shot up the golfer again, and again, and again, until he had administered the drug dose eight or 10 times, the shots encircling the lesion in a doughnut-shaped pattern around the nose and cheek. North noticed now that the feeling in the left side of his face was gone.

Snow picked up his instruments and began gently to carve off the lesion. North was not crazy about this routine, but he sat still. He knew how to do that because he had sat still for more than a few medical procedures in his 41 years. The bone disorder at age

12 that had him hopping around on crutches for a year-and-a-half. Bone spurs in his right elbow. A broken thumb, incurred in a 1986 fall that took him off the tour for three months. An injured right shoulder and a bone spur, removed from between the third and fourth vertebra on his neck, that wiped out the 1989 season. Not to mention six arthroscopic surgeries on his knees, five on the left, one on the right. North had sustained more injuries than most golfers—more, even, than most football players—and he knew the drill, knew you had to sit still while the doc made his moves. Mr. Cool, from head to toe. Only this deal was different from all the others that had come before. He'd never gone through anything like it, literally an in-your-face procedure.

Operating slowly, Snow cut away at the ala, moving in a circle, and pared away a tissue-thin sheet of skin from his nose. North remained conscious through the whole event, hyper-conscious even. Then Snow stripped away the epidermis and set the sample aside.

North headed home, still numb in the face, his nose heavily bandaged. Meanwhile, off went the tissue sample to the lab. North occupied himself at home, trying to go about his business—besides playing the sport, he designed golf courses and entertained executives on corporate golf outings—while a pathologist peered through a microscope studying the skin from his nose. North puttered around at his house. He checked his phone messages, planned his tournament schedule, made phone calls to keep in touch with clients. If the outer edges of the biopsy looked clean, free of the growth, then Snow had probably gotten it all. North wanted this to be a one-shot proposition, no encores, no curtain calls, just a doff of the cap on the 18th green and on to the next tournament. If, however, the sample was cancerous, North would have to haul himself back into the chair again, the same day, and Snow would once again do his stick-and-slice routine.

About two hours after the surgery ended, North called the lab to get the verdict. The sample had come back positive. He would have to go back in the afternoon for another session.

North climbed into his car and drove to the hospital. Snow repeated the procedure. Only this time, with the top layer of skin on his nose already peeled away, Snow injected anesthetic into the next level, a site already left raw and tender from the morning session. The surgeon pumped in another eight or 10 shots in a doughnut-shaped formation until the spot was adequately anesthetized. Then Snow resumed scraping away at the lesion on his nose, skinning it. It went slowly, gradual and measured and methodical, just like Andy lining up a recovery shot from the rough, and North was no more crazy about it in the afternoon than he had been in the morning. "I've never gone through pain like that," he recalled. "I've had all these other operations, on my elbow and my knees and my neck, but this was the worst. By far."

Within a half-hour, Snow had snipped off another swatch of skin from the nose to send as a sample to the pathology lab. North went home to wait—again—for the prognosis. He dabbled around in his office because he needed to do something with himself. Even so, he had to wonder how it would go this time. Twice under the knife in one day would be enough for him, thanks. He had planes to catch, tournaments to play, courses to design, prizes to win. Now it was 4:00 p.m., eight hours since he had first parked himself in that chair for the surgery. Time to phone the lab. So he called.

Again the biopsy came back positive.

"I thought this was going to be simple," North said. "Boy, was I wrong." Now he had to go back to Dr. Snow the next day. He had an appointment scheduled for more of the same.

❦ ❦ ❦

For centuries, most people avoided the sun unless they worked outdoors. Women would carry dainty parasols and wear hats and veils for protection. A lady of the aristocracy would whiten her face with finely ground flour, strictly for the sake of maintaining a regal pallor. Queen Elizabeth went so far as to lay milk-soaked strips of veal across her face for the same purpose.

Then, in the 1920s, the French fashion designer Coco Chanel began a revolution: she went to a party wearing a suntan. The guests, all of whom were fashionably pale, were shocked. By exposing her skin to sunlight, she had shattered an old taboo. Thanks to Chanel, a suntan came to be regarded as a symbol of ease and prosperity. Wearing a deep tan took on the same importance—especially for women—as putting on the right clothes, the right jewels and the right makeup.

Every summer thereafter, people stretched out in the warmth of the sunlight, surrendering themselves, half-naked and baby-like, to loll in the soothing rays. They smeared on the lotion, lay on blankets just so, and turned their bodies over and over, as if roasting on a spit. Then they went home believing they looked rich and healthy. Psychologists who have studied tanning habits suggest that people may possess a primal tanning instinct, an inborn compulsion to soak themselves in the sun. They point out that, to the devoted sunbather, the sun represents warmth and mother love; it comforts and enhances a sense of well-being.

Make no mistake: the quest for a deep, dark tan is still well-nigh epidemic, especially among devil-may-care teenagers. Earlier retirements, longer life expectancies, more extensive travel opportunities, and the population shift to the Sunbelt have kept the tan somewhat fashionable. A recent survey by the American Academy of Dermatology found that one-fourth of all adults surveyed take no precautions in the sun, one-third intentionally work on a tan, and fewer than half use sunscreens—even though 96 percent could name at least one negative effect of the sun, and 54 percent singled out the most serious danger, skin cancer.

Nobody—and nothing—outdoors escapes the effects of the sun. UV radiation can damage the body right down to its most basic components—proteins, enzymes, lipids, and DNA itself. UV light can penetrate lightweight summer clothing or wet T-shirts, and even affect those who swim underwater. As much as 80 percent of UV light can penetrate haze, light clouds, and fog. Rays also reflect upward off most surfaces, including sand, snow, ice, and water. Reflections from snow, in some instances, can increase sixfold the intensity of UV light. Temperature is much less critical a factor in skin damage from sun exposure than is commonly believed. Sunburn can occur just as easily on a winter day as on a summer day.

Let's say it's noon on a brilliantly sunny day. You're ready to take a quick lunch-time stroll, or plant tulip bulbs in your garden, or snooze on a bench in the local park. You think: No harm in getting just a little color, is there? Well, maybe there is. Psychiatrist Michael Pertschuck, director of the Center for Human Appearance at the University of Pennsylvania, found in a survey that most people view what he calls "incidental" tanning—sporadic instead of sustained, more casual than formal, often spontaneous rather than planned—with an attitude akin to nonchalance. Of 100 women age 40 or older, more than 75 percent thought that exposure of 15 to 60 minutes, during a certain time of day, was perfectly safe and acceptable.

But it's a mistake to assume that only prolonged exposure to the sun can damage your skin, Pertschuck says. "So what will forcibly bring home what is obviously still an unpalatable truth?" He asks. "It might help to think of the sun as a giant nuclear reactor. How much time would one want to bask in the glow of a nearby nuclear power plant? None. The same is true of the sun. There *is* no safe exposure."

❦ ❦ ❦

The Mohs surgery on the second day was even more difficult to endure. North showed up at the hospital at 8:00 a.m. and sat in the chair where it would all happen. Dr. Snow injected the anesthetic, once again eight to 10 shots in all, and sliced into the lesion, millimeter by millimeter, until he had another biopsy set to go under the microscope. North kept himself together, still Mr. Cool, and within 20 minutes, he was out of there.

"He's always met adversity matter-of-factly," Susan said. "He's very much the kind of guy who would rather not make a fuss out of anything. He was trying so hard to be so strong about it all. He was trying not to let me know he was in pain, that he could deal with it. But I knew. I could tell he was having a tough time. It was very hard on him, both physically and mentally. But it was hard on me, too, hard to see him in pain, watching him hurt."

Then Andy came home again to wait for word. Above all, through two days of surgical procedures, Andy North waited. After the first session, he waited to find out whether he needed a second, and after the second to see about a third, and now he waited yet again. He had too much time to think, same as with golf, and began to overevaluate his predicament. The operations at least kept him occupied, but they each lasted less than a half-hour, and then it was usually two hours before the lab report was ready, and another two before the next round of surgery. It was like being in that limbo between your first and second shots on, say, a par-four ninth hole. Which club would be best, the seven-iron or the eight? "Waiting around was agony for him," Susan said.

Thirty years earlier a doctor had told him about osteochondritis dissecans and limited his options when it came to playing sports. So it was now: he had little choice but to wait, no control at all over the situation, and as he waited, his anxiety and apprehension grew. "The waiting was definitely more traumatic than the operations themselves," North recalled. "The waiting and the wondering."

"How bad was the strain on us?" Susan said. "On a scale of one to 10, it went to 10. But you just do whatever you have to do to get you through those days. I did whatever I had to do to make Andy feel better, and he did the same for me. At the time you have no idea that it's taking a toll on you. You just need to do it and you zone out."

As it turned out, he had to go back. Again. This would make four surgeries within 36 hours. Four sessions of needles injected into his face, four sessions of cutting and scraping. The surgery he had originally shrugged off as hardly worth a second thought had turned into a big deal indeed. His face had grown tender from the insults of the hypodermic and the scalpel. The irony here was that in anesthetizing North to prevent pain, Snow caused plenty of it. The physician had no recourse now but to inject needles into the very sites he had already chiseled and excavated away, the sites now exposed and suppurating. Snow had no alternative, but to cut deeper into the nose, scraping off not just skin but cartilage and bone.

North knew that. He kept cool, even though he was concerned that the cancer might be worse than previously believed, that the surgery would leave his face—his handsome, son-of-a-Wisconsin-farmer's face—permanently disfigured. "Yeah, I was concerned, all right," he said. "Concerned and scared."

As Snow operated in the middle of his face for the fourth time, North felt his fear escalate to horror. "This turned into quite a huge mess," North recalled. "Vanity took over. It's my nose we're talking about. Snow had already cut off quite a bit of it. I'd looked in the mirror, under the bandages. There was almost nothing left to for him to take."

"Sure, it was traumatic," North said. "Any time a doctor starts carving up your face, you bet it's traumatic. How deep in my face could he go, and how big a hole would it make? I was at the end of my string. What would I look like after Snow finished carving? Was I going to lose my whole damn nose?"

By 1:30 p.m., Snow concluded his work, and two hours later, the pathologist, on examining the fourth biopsy in two days, reported that he had apparently succeeded in eliminating the cancerous growth. In the process, Snow had removed a section of nose the size of a quarter. "When we took off the bandages, I saw a big ugly hole on the side of my face," North said with a laugh. The damage came as no surprise to him.

"I saw his nose before he did," his wife said. "Dr. Snow asked us to look at it. Usually something like that does not bother me. But it's different when it's your own husband. I thought, 'How will they ever make this better?' A good portion of his nose and cheek were totally gone. It actually looked like somebody had put a big pair of pliers on the side of his nose and just pulled his whole nostril off. I mean, there was no nostril there. You could see bone and cartilage and blood. It looked like he had just come out of a terrible accident.

"Andy never said anything to me about how his nose looked."

Her husband considered himself lucky, justifiably so, certainly better off than other skin cancer patients he had seen outside, in the waiting room, the victims of sunlight with terrible scars, with noses and ears missing, with faces half burned away. That helped Andy keep it all in perspective. Besides, Dr. Snow assured the golfer that a plastic surgeon could repair his nose—"He is a man in the limelight and he was concerned about being left with a scar," the physician said—and North took him at his word.

❦ ❦ ❦

Only recently, in the last 20 years or so, have we discovered that a "healthy tan" is, in fact, a misnomer, a contradiction in terms. Vanity has begun losing out to health concerns as our attraction to the sun has become tempered with the knowledge that the sun is a health hazard and a tan is essentially a sign of cooked skin. Today, in the wake of these alarming warnings, many beachgoers have gone sun-shy. A recent Gallup survey found that fewer people described themselves as sunbathers than was the case five years earlier. Public opinion toward tanning—toward the idea that bronze is a badge of health and fitness—is going through a turnaround. This change of habit is occurring slowly across the board, virtually regardless of region, age, gender or income.

Yet fluorocarbons keep wearing down the ozone layer in the atmosphere, the natural shield against ultraviolet rays from the sun. As the ozone barrier thins, allowing more ultraviolet light to reach the earth undiluted, the rate of skin cancer may rise dramatically. The U.S. Environmental Protection Agency has predicted that by the year 2000, the ozone layer will erode roughly 5 percent, letting as much as 10 percent more radiation seep through to reach the earth and its five billion inhabitants. This breakdown could increase cases of malignant melanoma by 5 to 7 percent, basal-cell carcinoma by up to 10 percent, and squamous cell cancers by as much as 20 percent.

Parents, teachers and athletic coaches should educate children about sun exposure early while they're forming lifetime health habits. A study at Harvard recommended that the regular use of a sunscreen with an SPF 15 during the first 18 years of life could cut by 78 percent the risk of later developing skin cancer. Sunscreens filter the amount of ultraviolet rays from the sun that penetrate the skin and thereby retard burning and most other damage. Precautions are quick and easy. Apply sun care products liberally, at least 30 minutes before exposure to the sun, to allow the lotion to seep into the pores for maximum effectiveness.

Then make sure to reapply every hour or two, especially after heavy sweating or swimming.

To be extra careful, examine your skin—especially on the face—once a month to note any moles, blemishes, birthmarks or unusual growths. Check for changes in size, shape or color. If you see any differences, or if a sore fails to heal, see your physician without delay.

❦ ❦ ❦

On April 15, about a month after the wound on his face had healed to the satisfaction of all, North went to Dr. Syamasunder Rao, a plastic surgeon at the University of Wisconsin hospital. Dr. Rao performed reconstructive surgery, taking grafts of skin tissue from the back of his ears to rebuild his nose.

"I feel I'm really on the right track, and now it's going to be like starting all over again," North said at the time. "It would be nice if I could just go out and pick it up where I left off, but I'm sure it's going to be a struggle."

"It's all worked out very well," he recalled. "From a distance of more than 15 feet, it's hard for anyone to tell I've had any work done on my face, and that's nice. If you look for it up close, you can see a scar, but it's already fading away. Best of all, Dr. Snow says the affected area is healed and doing fine. It looks like we got this early and should have no other problems. I was fortunate we got this in time.

"I'm just glad my wife noticed."

Dr. Snow agreed: "Left untreated for a couple of years, he would've lost his entire nose."

In May 1991, after two months away from the PGA tour, North resumed his golf career. He played inconsistently, his knees and elbows still bothering him, all the questions about his nose distracting, but at least he went out and played, finishing 21 tournaments in 1991. "He's a very competitive individual, very conscientious," observed Dr. Snow. "All through the surgeries, he wanted to know everything in advance, so he could plan out everything."

"Andy would've succeeded, no matter what, even outside golf," said his wife. "For all I know, he might be running IBM today. His personality is such that he always wants to give it his best. When he plays tennis, he rushes the net and tries to kill the ball. When he does commentary for ESPN, he's always doing his homework rather than just winging it and taking it easy. Before a broadcast he looks through reference books and takes notes.

Whatever it is, he's either going to do it full-bore or not at all, never halfway."

In September 1991, the Wisconsin Division of the American Cancer Society designated North as its representative to send to Washington, D.C., for the 20th anniversary of the passage of the National Cancer Act. Each state picked a person to lobby Congress for a larger share of funding for cancer research.

"It's kind of ironic that, after working with the American Cancer Society for 15 years, all of a sudden I developed cancer myself," North said. "But I'm uneasy about being considered a survivor. It's hard for me to talk about this when I've had a little hunk of my nose cut off. It's hard to talk about surviving cancer when I'm fine and other people with cancer have lost arms and legs and are dying. What I've gone through is not a very big deal."

For years, he has worried about the sun harming his daughters Nichole, 18, who is very fair of skin and burns easily, and Andrea, 14. Both girls are sports-minded, partial to softball and bicycling, and like to be outdoors. As a result, North keeps sunscreen available for the family in every room of the house and in every car. He always reminds his daughters to take sunscreen on outings and forbids sunbathing at the beach, all in an effort to prevent another North from getting skin cancer.

"As far as sunscreens go, they never leave home without it," Susan said. "Our girls saw what he went through, and they were there for him. They saw Andy accepted it, so they accepted it. Never any panic. They're made from the same mold and followed his lead. But just recently they decided they'd had enough of his constant reminders. They said to me, 'Mom, please tell Dad we put on our sunscreens and wear our hats. There's no need for him to tell us anymore.'"

"Unfortunately, most of the damage is done when you're a kid," said Andy, who still goes twice a year for skin checkups. "I did a good job covering up in the sun over the last 15 years, but for the first 25, man, I was out of control."

Largely because of North—he clearly had the worst case of skin cancer in pro golf—more golfers now take precautions, applying sunscreen and donning hats. Coppertone signed a deal with the PGA tour as its official sunscreen product. Centinela Hospital of Los Angeles provides the tour with a trailer that goes from tournament to tournament providing both sun-care prevention and treatment. More golfers avoid the peak-exposure hours between 10:00 a.m. and 2:00 p.m., and instead practice in either early morning or late evening, when sunlight is at its mildest.

While he continued to play 15 to 20 golf tournaments a year, North remained committed to the mission of educating others about the importance of early detection for skin cancer. "Now that I've gone through this, I drive by the beach and see all these people laying out there, trying to get as brown as they can," he said. "It's hard to believe people still do that stuff. They're cooking themselves. Thousands and thousands of people get skin cancer every year and get treated for it and die from it. The numbers are shocking and unbelievable. People should just avoid the sun as much as possible and get themselves checked regularly. It's so easy."

"The sun is like anything else in life," he said. "Too much of anything can cause problems. Cars are wonderful, too—as long as you remember not to jump out in front of one. You just have to be careful out there."

Chapter 7

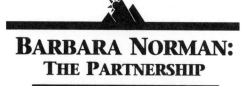

BARBARA NORMAN:
THE PARTNERSHIP

Let's go, Barbara Norman thought. Let's go already. It was 7:00 a.m., 45 minutes after sunrise on October 14, 1989. The day had dawned cool, about 75 degrees, under clear skies stippled by cirrus clouds in Kailua-Kona, Hawaii, an island of volcanoes and molten lava simmering at 2,000 degrees. More than 1,250 athletes from around the world, amateur and professional, had waded into the bay off Kailua Pier, the starting line for the Bud Light Ironman Triathlon World Championship. The athletes ranged in age from 18 to 75, hailed from 48 U.S. states and 49 countries, and would need between nine and 17 hours to complete the race.

Let's get going here, thought Norman. A handsome woman, she has high, chiseled cheekbones, deep-set, ice-blue eyes and light brown hair streaked with blond highlights and pulled back tight in a ponytail. Wearing an orange bathing cap, black-and-white swim goggles, and a black-and-pink swimsuit, she stood waist-deep in Kailua Bay stretching her torso from side to side. An official with a waterproof black pen had marked her biceps and outer thighs with race identification number 841. On the beach, behind the competitors, the fronds of the coconut palm trees swayed in the early morning breeze. Race pennants festooned over the water flapped softly. The water was warm, about 79 degrees, and salty and clear. The bay was transparent straight to the bottom, and some swimmers later sighted schools of dolphins and manta rays fishtailing along 40 feet below the surface.

An official fired a small cannon to signal the start of the contest. Boom! All the competitors plunged in headfirst for the 2.4-mile swim out of the harbor and back. We've started! Norman rejoiced. Like a teeming school of fish, the swimmers churned the bay into foaming white water. They swam parallel to Alii Drive and turned around at the buoy at the Kona Tiki, then headed back to the pier.

The 51-year-old Greenwich, Connecticut, attorney had trained long and hard for this, her first Ironman. She had come far to reach this starting line, farther than most of her competitors would ever know. The average racer in the event trains for 18 to 24 hours a week, for a total of about eight months; a weekly regimen typically consists of seven miles of swimming, 175 miles of bicycle riding and 48 miles of running—and, just for good measure, such cross-training activities as weight lifting, yoga, stretching, and calisthenics. With such intense preparation under her belt, Norman felt her anxiety slowly evaporate.

She was among the oldest competitors in the race, one of 16 entrants in the 50- to 54-year-old group. Norman broke comfortably into her stroke, with the attitude that age is largely immaterial. She felt totally happy, with one minor exception. In the madcap rush, other swimmers tended to barrel ahead, regardless of obstacles, and some kicked and crawled right over fellow contestants, including her.

Finishing the swim, Norman breathed heavily, her arms and shoulders sore from stroking, then climbed out of the harbor and headed toward the 1,250-odd bicycles lined up on the pier. One event down, two to go. The bicycle ride in the Ironman is 112 miles long, about half the distance between New York City and Boston. That morning, Norman had pumped the tires on her bicycle to the proper air pressure and set the gears for the ride, to cut down on the time spent in transition from the swim. Now she quickly donned her hot-pink helmet (to match her swim suit). She strapped onto herself a "fanny-pack" containing cut-up Power Bars and pedaled off near the middle of the racers. She headed up the steep hill and turned north through the intersection at Palani Road and Queen Kaahumanu Highway—known to the locals and diehard triathletes as the "Queen K." Pumping away, her head lowered to cut wind resistance, Norman sped through the town and out toward the lava fields against a soundtrack of clicking gears and the hornet-like buzzing of speeding bicycle wheels.

About three miles into the race, Norman started to feel a sharp pain in her left foot, as if she might have pulled a muscle. She forced herself to stop thinking about the pain for the next 20 miles, but soon it radiated along her leg, growing severe. Now she glanced down at her left foot, about to take off the shoe for a close look. There, still wedged in the back of her shoe, was a shoehorn. In her haste to climb aboard her bike and start rolling, she had forgotten to take it out of her shoe. And in her zeal to put some miles behind her, she had biked 25 miles with a shoehorn eating into the sole of her foot.

The shoehorn removed, Norman rode north along the Kona coast, skirting the Pacific Ocean, her immediate destination the turn-around point at Hawi. She pedaled along the Queen K, past flat lava fields and rolling hills. The lava flats are made up of black lava rock scorched by the sun. It's a desolate moonscape, pockmarked with craters, spooky and hypnotic and otherworldly. It seemed endless to her. Ironman competitors report that bicycling across this stretch offers the sensation of moving without actually getting anywhere. It's as if one is pedaling in place while the panorama, like a movie set, is scrolling past with metronomic monotony.

By midmorning, the temperature had climbed to 100 degrees, with humidity hovering around 90 percent. The heat radiated from the highway, shimmering in the air, the asphalt baking in the sun. The heat was the heaviest challenge. Norman fueled herself at the turn-around with cans of Exceed, a complex-carbohydrate nutritional supplement, and bananas. (Before the day was out, she would burn an estimated 6,000 to 12,000 calories and lose roughly 10 pounds.)

Norman leaned her head forward, her forearms pressed against the handlebars, throttling downhill, going faster now, hitting 45 miles per hour. It could get tricky flirting with the frontiers of human endurance in this kind of environment. One highly touted competitor, her potassium levels lowered by dehydration, crashed her bicycle into a parked car. She broke her neck and, though not paralyzed, needed to wear a neck brace for the next five months.

Norman stopped her bike in Keahou, at the Kona Surf Resort, and got off to pick up the next leg of the triathlon: the marathon, all 26 miles and 385 yards of it. Two events down, one to go. She showered first, quickly, and slipped on her running shoes, again with her trusty shoehorn, only this time she remembered to yank it out of her sneaker before bolting off. She headed along Alii Drive again, zigzagged along Hualalai Road, and passed through Kailua Village via the Kuakini Highway. She took short strides, barely lifting her feet off the ground. The water bottle weighed heavily on her back. She stripped it off and, passing the house she had rented with family and friends, tossed it into the bushes. It seemed like forever before she passed Keahole Airport and turned around to go back for the second half of the run.

At 6:20 p.m.—nearly half a day after Norman had plunged into the water—the sun dipped below the horizon, and Norman was still making tracks. As a jeweled curtain of night draped the sky, a race volunteer handed glowsticks to her and other competitors to carry through the cooling Hawaiian dusk. Norman had felt strong until this point, but now she realized she had overtrained. She ran slowly now, just for the sake of maintaining some movement. Some racers slowed to a walk and shambled along the roadside. Norman stopped running, too, walking a few steps at each of the water stops spaced at one-mile intervals along the course. The lights from oncoming cars on the Kuakini Highway flashed brightly in her eyes. She felt herself starting to run out of steam, her quadriceps screaming in protest at the concussive abuse of the hardtop pavement. She wished the race were over.

Norman ran the last few miles in almost pitch dark, the stars brilliant in the South Pacific canopy of night overhead. From a distance she spotted the lights over Kona at the finish line and felt in her heart a pulse of excitement. Her whole family had come—her mother, her two sisters Janice and Mary Lou, and her daughter Kathleen. Her friend and training partner Kathy Salvo, a fellow competitor now ahead of her in the race, would also be there at the finish line, cheering her on. She came round the crowd-lined Alii Drive, running downhill. She had just wanted to finish, however slow her pace, whatever her final time or standing. But now, with the crowd rooting her on, she found herself running faster and faster. Even 13 hours into the race, the crowd stood foursquare behind the competitors. Just then a bystander yelled to Norman, "You look wonderful. You can do it! Keep going!" And she all but sprinted the last half-mile down toward the pier.

She crossed the finish line, smiling, and her family swarmed around her, kissing and congratulating her. She had finished the Ironman in 13:14:18, third in her age group. Her finish symbolized the completion of a personal odyssey infinitely more grueling than a single triathlon. In the two years before the race, Norman had sustained grave hardships back to back. First she had lost her beloved husband to a congenital medical defect. Then a physician had diagnosed her with breast cancer.

The night after the triathlon, at an awards banquet ceremony, Norman was honored for her third-place age-group finish. She was presented with an Ironman Timex watch that says: "Kona, Hawaii, October 14, 1989." She still wears the watch today, but no watch could express the strides she's made.

❦ ❦ ❦

"When I was in my late 20s and my daughter Kathleen was a baby," says Norman, "I would do light exercise. Calisthenics. Deep knee bends. Toe touching. That kind of stuff. I would also do some gardening. We had a garden about 25 yards long in our back yard. I must have planted every vegetable imaginable. Potatoes, tomatoes, lettuce, carrots, peas, corn, string beans. When Kathleen was about 6, I started swimming laps two or three times a week at the local Y. First I swam a quarter-mile, then a half, then three-quarters. Finally, I could swim a whole mile. I always liked swimming.

"Later on, I got serious about golf—my first husband played a lot of golf. The golf course was only about a mile from our house. Every day, I played either nine or 18 holes, or hit a couple of buckets. I took lessons, too, and got pretty good. I usually scored between 90 and 100. I played in some club tournaments and won a few championships. But golf was a poor sport for me because I'm very intense. I concentrated too hard, without chatting much. You have to be relaxed and easygoing to play golf well. I never thought golf was fun, really. I took it so seriously that I often left the golf course in tears. I needed something else.

"I started running around our neighborhood in 1978, shortly after I got divorced and graduated from Fordham University School of Law. I was 40 years old. I wanted to run mainly to relieve the tension of working at a New York City law firm. I had to take the pressure off myself. I found that I needed exercise in the morning, before I got on the train to Manhattan, to mellow myself out, to keep me from feeling so uptight and nervous at the office. But I also had an ulterior motive for taking up running.

"My obstetrician–gynecologist, Parke Gray, would run around the neighborhood, too, right past my house. Parke was tall, slim, and good-looking. He had fine smooth skin and strong hands with long fingers, perfect for a surgeon. Like me, he was also divorced. And he lived only a couple of blocks away. I decided it might be good for us to have a common pursuit such as running around the neighborhood. I expected that he might then think of me as a jock.

"We started running together—and dating—in the fall of 1978. On my first run with Parke, we ran down to the Belle Haven section of town, and it was hilly. We were going up a hill, and I was dying. He said, 'You just follow the person ahead of you and watch his feet and do the same with your feet.' So as we went up this hill, I watched his feet in front of me. And I was ready to die. We ran a loop about five or six miles around. It was hard, very uncomfortable, and I really disliked it. But I never admitted that to Parke. It was a new challenge, and running was very much in vogue then. I was serious about it and read all the Jim Fixx books. It was a kind of courtship.

"Parke and I got married in 1979. It later turned out that he had started running only to impress *me*, and soon after we got married, he stopped."

Norman leans back on a sofa in the living room of her summer home in Montauk, on the furthermost tip of Long Island. A Massachusetts native, she speaks with clipped authority, a vestige of New England in her voice. The room is airy, with arched windows facing a deck, each window like a frame for the ocean beyond. The bookshelves and coffee table reveal copies of *Triathlete* magazine, the *New York Times,* a few John Updike novels. The three-bedroom house she owns rests on a bluff jutting out near some sand dunes that overlook a choppy expanse of the Atlantic Ocean. On the beach, strewn with shells and sunbathers, reeds rustle in the stiff breeze and sand crabs scuttle along.

"But for me, the running took on a life of its own," Norman said. "Another local doctor who ran, Sherman Bull, came up to me at a party and said, 'Now that you're running, you really should enter this five-mile race coming up.' It was a Sri Chinmoy Race in Old Greenwich. Sherman had the idea that, if you ran, you should always enter races because it gave meaning to your training. I had never considered myself to be in training, but I liked the sound of that idea, the idea that I was in training and acting like a real athlete. That five-mile race was hard work, and I had dry heaves at the end. But I finished it, and I ran another race, and then another, all five- and six-mile races.

"In 1981 Sherman was running in the New York City Marathon, and his wife Peggy and I drove there from Connecticut to sit in the stands and watch him and all the marathoners coming across the finish line. The announcer would call out the name of the finisher, and the crowd would yell and cheer, and the runner would wave or just smile, or both. But it was not the well-known marathoners—who were obviously in wonderful condition and who were not suffering any discomfort—who most impressed me. It was those who were truly extending themselves with this effort, going beyond what they might ordinarily be capable of doing, especially the handicapped runners. They impressed me a lot.

"What stood out for me was one guy who was disabled. It was hard for him to finish, he was hobbling so much, but when he came across the line, the crowd was so proud of him, and you could see he was so happy. He was just so proud of himself. He struck me as very courageous. It was moving and emotional and exciting for me, seeing people like him, so exhausted but still overcoming those obstacles, and seeing that the running, the finishing, had brought such happiness. I had tears coming down my face. Watching Alberto Salazar would not have made me cry like that.

"And I got an idea. I'd seen people finishing after five hours, people who seemed to be in the same kind of shape as I was. I thought, Gee, maybe I can do a marathon. So that prospect excited me, and when I got home I said to Parke, 'I think I'll start training for next year's marathon.' I'm not sure he believed me. I had some doubts myself for a long time. I'd never even run seven miles, and yet here I was thinking about covering more than 26 miles. But I figured I had a whole year to get ready.

"The next day I went out and ran around the Field Point Circle section of Greenwich. By July or August of that year, I could do 20 miles and I knew I was going to finish the New York City Marathon. It was just a question of how fast—or how slow, as the case may be—and I remember being concerned that it would take me forever."

Norman need hardly have felt such concern. In the New York City Marathon in October of 1982, she trod along with 16,000 other runners and finished with a highly respectable 3:51 effort. As she reflects in her living room on this early performance, Norman looks rather like an astronaut. She wears a sleeveless tan running shirt, her arms sinewy, her face tawny from year-round training. With her eyes set deep under a formidable brow, she gives the impression, only half-true, of staring intently. She also conveys, probably without meaning to, an image of Yankee rectitude, as if she regards any form of idleness, at least in herself, with well-nigh Puritanical intolerance.

She went on to race in other marathons, she said, first in Stamford, Connecticut, then in Washington, D.C. But soon she developed sciatic pain, brought on, her doctors surmised, by a herniated disk in her fourth lumbar vertebra, the result of a 20-year-old laminectomy.

"It was like a toothache running down my whole leg, right down to my toes," Norman said. "It hurt all the time—when I ran, when I drove, even just from putting my foot on the brake."

She decided that was it—no more marathons. Quitting would mean she could stop running 55 miles a week, and maybe she could try a more well-rounded event, involving swimming and cycling, but less running. I know, she thought. Next year, I'll do a triathlon. Originally, she had thought that triathletes were nuts. "Then I realized, crazy as it sounds, that triathlons would actually be easier on my back and legs—like a form of treatment."

She enlisted in her first triathlon, the Montauk Triathlon, in June of 1983. But the event was full and her application was rejected. Norman called the director of the race, Bob Aaron, to say she was going out to Montauk anyway. She said to Aaron, "I've already trained, I've got a hotel room, and I have to do this race or my husband will kill me. He's a doctor and he's canceled his office hours and reshuffled his appointments a month ahead of time so we could go out to Montauk together."

Aaron said, "I'm sorry, Barbara, but the race is full. There's nothing I can do."

"Are you sure?" she said.

Aaron paused and said, "Well, maybe if someone cancels, we can make room for you."

Norman recalled: "So Parke and I went out to Montauk on a Thursday, about a three-hour drive, and on Friday, the day before the race, I went up to the registration table and introduced myself to Aaron. He said nobody had canceled and he still had no room for me. I said, 'Gosh, I'm here anyway, so I'll just have to wait until someone does cancel.' And he just said, 'Okay, we'll see.' And he tried to ignore me for about a half-hour. But then he probably thought, I've got to get rid of this leech. She's starting to bug me. So he said, 'Okay, come here, I'll give you an entry form,' and he handed me the form. I would have stayed there all night. That's just my approach.

The Montauk Triathlon entailed the international or Olympic distance: a 1.5-kilometer swim (about a mile) across a lake, a 40-kilometer bike ride (about 25 miles) and a 10-kilometer run (about 6.2 miles). Most other competitors owned sleek, lightweight, customized racing bicycles from France or Italy, worth at least $1,000 apiece; Norman went with a bike once owned by her daughter, complete with kickstand and book rack, a vehicle valued at about $100 at best. Norman finished the race first in the 40-49 age group.

In her next contest, the Mighty Hamptons Triathlon in Southampton, Norman rode a new, decidedly adult racing bike. But she gave another obvious hint of her newcomer status. "I was riding my bike, and I went over a bump and my bifocals went flying," she said. "I actually stopped the bike in the middle of the race, with the other bikes speeding past me. I got off and went back on the track to pick my glasses off the ground. Then I walked back and climbed back onto my bike. If that happened today, I would just say to myself, 'Too bad about those glasses,' and keep on riding. Just shows how my attitude about competition has changed." Even detained by this unexpected pit stop, Norman ran third among her 40- to 49-year-old contemporaries.

"I never tried in the early years to beat anyone, never cared about coming in ahead of other racers," she said. "Sometimes near the finish line a woman would sprint past me, and I would let her go. I would think, Who cares? This is no big deal. I disliked the pressure of trying to beat someone; that was too much like my experience on the golf course. I competed only with myself, to try to get the best time. When I started competing in marathons and triathlons, I considered myself a winner if all I ever did was finish a race."

She qualified for the Hawaiian Ironman in 1984, then again in 1985, 1987, and 1988, but opted to abstain. She felt the need to acquire some serious competitive seasoning before venturing to Hawaii. In the meantime, the switch from marathons to triathlons registered a therapeutic effect, and the sciatica in her legs never bothered her again.

From the outset, Barbara and Parke turned these athletic outings into romantic occasions. As at her first triathlon, in Montauk, the couple would book a room in a quiet inn near the race site, whether East Hampton or Cape Cod, and drive there together for a three-day weekend. The day before the event, she and Parke would loll around a beach, snacking, or go see some sights, then have a gourmet dinner, wine included. The race never really topped the agenda—it was an excuse to get away. Parke, for that matter, never took much of an interest in triathlons. Over these long, leisurely dinners away from Greenwich, he and Barbara talked about anything and everything—except the race to come.

❦ ❦ ❦

In 1980, Parke suffered a grand-mal seizure. He and Barbara were shopping at a supermarket when he told her he felt ill and sensed something serious coming on. As Barbara drove her husband to a hospital in Greenwich, he went into the seizure. "I had no idea what was happening," she said. "He was having convulsions and it was so frightening. I drove at breakneck speed, thinking it might be a heart attack, praying out loud. I thought, Dear God, don't let anything happen to this man."

At the hospital, the convulsions subsided and, suddenly, Parke was okay. Doctors later found, via CAT scan, that Parke had a congenital condition, a malformation of blood vessels in the brain, known as arteriovenous malformation (AVM). The diagnosis meant, in the simplest possible terms, that Parke had blood vessels so knotted together that someday one vessel would burst and he would hemorrhage, probably fatally. The seizure was a portent. The prognosis was that, within a few years—no one could say with any accuracy how many—he would be either disabled or dead.

Parke went to a clinic in Canada to inquire about surgery. When he came back, he said to Barbara, "Look, I've decided surgery isn't a viable solution. We're not going to talk about it. We're just going to put it out of our minds. It's always possible that nothing will happen for a while."

Still, Barbara encouraged her husband to undergo the surgery. But Parke would have none of it. "He would say to me, 'Well, what if I'm incapacitated by the surgery and you have to take care of me?'" she recalled. "I knew the surgery was risky. He might end up the same as a stroke victim. He wanted to avoid being disabled and having to give up his medical practice. He was afraid the operation would impair his memory. He once said to me, 'What if I have trouble remembering who you are?' Once he determined that his disorder was inoperable, we just tried to put it out of our minds. He really did think that this was not going to happen to him, at least not for a long time. Some people with the condition live 20 years, and we hoped that he would be among those people.

"We had brief bouts of depression about his condition. We would get maudlin and I would say, 'I would never want to go on living without you.' But then Parke would say, 'Look, neither of us is in control of what's going to happen to us. No sense in worrying or being anxious about something beyond our control. All we can control is our relationship.'

"I never could put it out of my mind, not for a single day," Barbara said. "Every morning when I would run up the driveway, I would see him sitting in this red reclining chair in the sun room reading the *New York Times*. I'd wave to him and he'd always wave back. Every day, as I went out for my run, it occurred to me that something might have happened to him. It was always a gnawing little worry in the back of my head. Always wondering whether he would still be there in the sun room to wave when I got back."

Parke and Barbara had planned a one-week vacation in late January of 1987. One morning about two weeks before the vacation, Parke woke up at around 5:00 a.m., moaning. Barbara turned on the night table lamp to look at him and immediately saw the symptoms of a hemorrhage in progress. Parke was unable to speak or move his right side. She said, "Oh, Parke, shall I call an ambulance?"

He nodded his head yes.

"Oh, Parke, I love you so," she said. She saw her husband had tears in his eyes. "But by the time I called the ambulance a minute or two later, I think he was already gone," she said. "It was not a bad way to die. A very quick, really easy death."

Barbara thinks often and warmly about her late husband, drawing fortitude from his example. "I think he just trusted in God," she said. "He had a lot of faith, and was never frightened about anything. He would say, 'We just have to leave it up to God to do whatever He's going to do with our lives. Let's not worry about it. We'll just let the Good Lord decide when it's my time and you'll do what has to be done when it comes.' And through him, I trusted that everything was going to be all right.

"In the eight years Parke and I were married, we were very much in love, very happy together. We just focused on being together, and our relationship was wonderful. We resolved, after his condition was diagnosed, to live our lives as normally as possible. If his death taught me any lesson at all, it's that you have to live the best possible life together, no matter what.

"I remember Parke would sometimes say to me, 'I wish you would stop doing so much of this racing.' And I would say to him, 'Look, if anything happens to you, I'm going to be very unhappy. I'm probably going to be a wreck. If anything happens to you—if you're incapacitated or dead—I'm going to need something to take my mind off my unhappiness. It's going to be important for me to have this sport. Being able to go out and run and bike and swim and sign up for a race is going to be very helpful to me.'

"It turned out I was right."

❦ ❦ ❦

Norman had begun at age 40 to perform monthly self-examination of her breasts, as a precaution against breast disease. She would go into the shower, apply soap to her hand to heighten the sensitivity of her nerve endings, and run her fingers over the contours of her bosom. After all, her husband was a gynecologist. He encouraged her to religiously practice these preventive measures against cancer. But Barbara needed no extra pressure from Parke. Even before meeting him, she had initiated a dutiful habit of going in regularly for an equally valuable precaution, a mammogram. At first, she underwent the X-rays every few years, then, as she neared 40, she switched to annual tests.

The week after Parke died, Norman checked herself in the

shower, as per her monthly schedule. And, for the first time in her life, she felt something on her left breast, below the nipple. It felt soft and when she pressed it, it would give. She thought, Have I had this lump before?

"Then I got these morbid feelings," she said. "I'd lived for eight years with this man I'd loved so much and now he was gone."

And now she thought, This is it. I'm going to die from breast cancer. I'll be with Parke and that'll be great.

"I actually thought that," she recalled. "That this breast cancer was going to kill me and I'd be with my husband. It was in the back of my mind that I would let the breast cancer become a kind of suicide—and that dying would reunite me with my husband. Pretty depressing. But then, my mind was totally shot from mourning Parke, just a jumble of thoughts. I argued with myself about what to do."

What Norman decided, in the grip of this death wish, was to let this discovery go. Her grief over Parke was still so fresh that she adamantly refused to think about, much less do anything about, the lump on her left breast. It was as if a jolt of electroshock had erased the issue from her memory. "I would just let the cancer take me," she said.

In April of 1987, when Norman was sitting at the locker of her Greenwich swim club, she met Kathy Bambace-Salvo, also an avid swimmer. Salvo sidled over to Norman and said, "I'm going to sign up for the Cape Cod Endurance Race next year. Want to do it with me?" The Cape Cod event, which would be held in October the next year, was the equivalent of a full-fledged Ironman triathlon, more race than Norman had ever taken on to that point.

"No," Norman said, "I'm not going to do anything like that. But I'll train with you."

Salvo was 23, the same age as Norman's daughter Kathleen. A pretty, young woman, short and compact, with sturdy legs and broad shoulders, Salvo had a head of glossy black hair and perfectly straight white teeth. Married and a resident of nearby Stamford, Connecticut, she worked as a stockbroker with Paine Webber in the fast-paced, high-adrenaline atmosphere of Wall Street. She had just taken up triathlons and needed an experienced training partner.

And so, despite a 26-year age difference, Barbara began to train with Salvo. At first, the arrangement was ad hoc. Salvo would call Norman and say, "Come on, let's go for a bike ride." That summer, they logged progressively longer and longer distances, cycling for 20, 30, 40 miles. By Labor Day, they had completed what's called a century, 100 miles in one shot, a first for both.

"I always found it so funny that she would invite me on bike trips with her and her young friends," Norman said. "I think she must have felt a little sorry for me."

The rigorous training regimen with Kathy turned out, quite unexpectedly, to be a balm for Barbara. "I had to do something physical, to take my mind off my troubles," Norman said. "I was terribly unhappy, mostly about Parke, but also about the lump. I thought all the time about both these disasters. So I would exercise even more than usual. Kathy and I would run six or seven or eight miles. We would swim and cycle, too. The exercise enabled me to sleep very well at night, and the better I rested, the better I functioned at work. I just stayed with my routine, and my workouts with Kathy became the most important aspect of my day.

"A game of chess would not have done the job, nor would reading or painting or volunteer work," she said. "No matter how I felt about losing the man I was in love with, the exercise gave me a sense of well-being and happiness. I would feel good. Happy. Upbeat. It definitely had to be something physical to pull me through. And somewhere in there, for the first time, I started believing in endorphins. After Parke died, the running was absolutely like a medication for me, an anesthetic for the pain. The training with Kathy helped me get through my period of mourning."

But now eight months had passed since the suspect growth on her breast had aroused her concern. All through her tandem training with Kathy, Barbara had thought, Well, as soon as I finish this next race, I'll have this lump taken out.

"Now we're talking about eight whole months since I'd noticed the lump on my breast," she said. "I realized that when you have a lump, you have to go to a doctor." I said to myself, 'Well, this is ridiculous. Eight months is a long time to wait.' No woman with a lump in her breast should ever wait as I long as I did. Or wait at all, for that matter. Besides, I don't believe in suicide, and if Parke had been there, he would have disapproved. I thought, This is just the wrong idea. I better go have it checked out. I decided that if you have something wrong with you, going without seeing a doctor is irresponsible. I love my daughter, and it would have been unfair to her if I let something bad happen to me."

Norman went for her yearly physical at a New York City cancer center and seized the opportunity to point out her lump to a gynecologist. He performed a mammogram, along with a hands-on exam, and a few days later informed her, in writing, that he had found nothing worrisome. But somehow Norman doubted his word. She sought a second opinion, and scheduled an appointment with Dr. Sherman Bull, the surgeon who had originally recommended the marathon to her.

She said to Sherman, "Take a look at this lump and tell me what you think."

After a close look, Sherman said, "Well, it looks like nothing. But if you want, we'll take it out. It's only going to get bigger, so we might as well remove it."

"Fine," she said. "When do you want to schedule it?"

"Let's take it out after the Christmas holidays," Sherman said.

Though Norman intended to go along with this plan, she saw yet another gynecologist in the meantime, for a third opinion. He, too, said, "No need to worry about that lump." But he also issued a warning: "You should have it taken out," he added, "because it may mask a cancerous lump underneath."

It was agreed, then, that Norman would go to Sherman in January 1988 for surgery to remove the lump. She had competed all through 1987, in 12 races altogether—five triathlons, as well as marathons and biathlons. But then, due to a scheduling conflict, the January appointment was canceled.

Norman said to Sherman, "Does it matter whether I have the lump taken out now? Or can I wait until after my training season in the fall?"

"No," Sherman said, "I see no problem with putting it off. We can do that if you want. The only risk is that the lump will get bigger."

"Well," Norman said, "what's the difference if my scar is an inch long or an inch-and-a-half? Let's put it off, because if I have the lump taken out now, I'll have to stop swimming for three weeks."

All three doctors Norman had consulted by this point had, in effect, told her not to worry. Put it off she would—at her peril, unbeknown to her.

In 1988 Barbara and Kathy began training seriously for the Cape Cod Endurance Race. Kathy would meet Barbara at her Greenwich home at 5:00 a.m. to run, swim or bike for two hours. After work, in the evening, they would meet again for a one-hour session, this time adding a weight-lifting routine to the program. On Saturdays, they trained for six hours; on Sundays, another six.

In the summer, Barbara sketched out a chart to detail her training schedule almost down to the last decimal point. As she neared major competitions, she would chronicle her progress on a chart taped to her kitchen door. Each day she set a goal for the mileage she wished to log in running, swimming, and bicycling, then jotted down her record. She never let herself get away with shortcuts. One week in late June, she planned to run 30 miles; instead, she racked up 17.5 miles—and the chart so stated in no uncertain terms. Even where the disparity between intention and accomplishment was hair-splitting, Norman prided herself on fidelity to fact. During another week in mid-July, she had expected to cover 34 miles; as she noted in her training chart, she managed to accumulate only 33, a mere mile less.

She trained every day, with the exception of several breaks in late August for the sake of tapering, a means of winding down to rest and let the muscles heal before a major event. The program intensified from late June to late August, during which time she increased her weekly running workload from 30 miles to 40, her bicycling from 105 miles to 200, and her swimming from 8,000 yards to 11,000. Through the summer, Barbara was on a hot streak, claiming two first-place and two second-place finishes in her age group in triathlons in, respectively, Baltimore, Rhode Island, Chicago, and South Carolina.

Her race season culminated in September, at the Cape Cod Endurance Race in Hyannis, Massachusetts. Ten days before the race, Barbara and Kathy rented a house in Cape Cod. Taking nothing for granted, they practiced on the marathon course for the race—six miles along this stretch one day, another six along a different section the next.

Despite this preparation, Barbara turned to Kathy the day before the event and said, "I feel sick. I'm not going to do well in this race. I may not be able to finish."

Kathy had seen Barbara pull this routine before. Before a race, Barbara always got butterflies and sometimes threatened, rather dramatically, that she might be too sick to race. It was similar to a child with a case of nerves asking her mother for permission to stay home from school. "I usually think it's pretty funny," Kathy recalled, "so I just laughed."

The race began at 7:00 a.m.; Barbara and Kathy hugged and kissed each other at the starting line. The partners planned to finish the race together, something they had never done before. After the bicycle ride, Kathy led by a half hour. Then, around the 14th mile of the marathon, Barbara caught up with her. Kathy felt lousy and had nothing left in her gas tank. As Barbara slowed down alongside her, Kathy said to her, "No, no, go on."

Barbara would have none of it. "We're going to finish this race together," she insisted. I'm going to walk with you if I have to."

"No, no, go on," Kathy pleaded again.

"I'm not going for any world record," Barbara reminded her. "What difference does it make?"

"Please go," Kathy said with a grimace. Then, good-naturedly, she added, "You're bothering me."

With that, Barbara went ahead, alone, the oldest racer in the event. And, after more than half a day of strenuous and uninterrupted physical exertion, she finished the Cape Cod Endurance Race in 12:25:02, finishing first among those 40 years of age and older. But that's not all. Notwithstanding her earlier remark to Kathy—to wit: "I'm not going for any world record"— Barbara had, in fact, established a new triathlon world record for an Ironman distance race in her age group. She had shattered the previous record by more than half an hour.

But her jubilation was short-lived, because she decided the time had come for her to stop playing Russian roulette. In November she at last went to Dr. Bull to take care of the lump in her left breast. "I'd waited all this time because doctors had told me I had a good lump," she said. "But no lump is a good lump. If you have a lump in your breast, you have it taken out. By this time we're talking about almost two years since I'd noticed it. That kind of wait can kill some women."

She entered St. Joseph's Hospital in Stamford for the long-delayed lumpectomy to remove the growth. Sherman took her into an anteroom and told her the operation would last only five minutes. He said it would be like taking off a wart. Barbara lay on the operating table, and he gave her an injection of Novocain. Sherman chatted about his marathon running and his mountain-climbing adventures. All quite casual, quite friendly.

Then he sliced a small incision in her left breast.

"Suddenly, he got quiet," Barbara recalled. "I knew right then and there what I had. No need to get a slide back from a pathologist."

Barbara looked at him and said, "Sherman, you're awfully quiet. You got bad news there? Does it look bad?"

"Yeah," Sherman said, "it's very bad." The physician extracted a microscopic tissue sample to serve as a biopsy and briskly sewed up the incision. He left the room and gave the sample to a pathologist. Then he came back in and delivered the message Barbara most feared hearing.

"Well," Sherman said, "you have breast cancer."

❦ ❦ ❦

One in nine. Those are the odds that a woman in the United States will develop breast cancer during her lifetime, according to the American Cancer Society. In the last half-century, this disease has more than doubled in incidence in the United States, leaping from a ratio of 1-to-20 back in 1940. Every 15 minutes an American woman hears the diagnosis: "You have breast cancer." Women develop breast cancer more than any other single form of cancer. The disease annually attacks 180,000 American women and, in an estimated 46,000 cases, leads to death. Breast cancer is also the second major cause of all cancer deaths: One out of four women who get it die from it.

But women can significantly reduce those risks. Breast cancer, if discovered early—before its symptoms can be perceived by the touch of a hand—can be cured in 9 of 10 cases. The agenda? Number one: breast self-examination. Number two: physician checkup. Number three: a mammogram.

Simple.

But it's not happening, at least not nearly enough, and certainly not with any technical proficiency. All too many women refrain from self-examination, consultation with a physician, and mammography. A recent survey revealed, for example, that although 89 percent of women know about monthly breast self-examination, only 53 percent do it. Another study showed that only 8 percent of women *correctly* perform breast self-examination. As for X-ray tests, the National Cancer Institute finds that only about 30 percent of women over 40 years old have regular mammograms—and 35 percent have never had even one. Indeed, about 18 million women today regularly go in for the procedure, but about 34 million other women—some four million of whom are at high risk for breast cancer—steer clear. One study of breast cancer showed that fewer than half of the cases diagnosed were caught before the tumors had spread to the lymph nodes.

Why do so many millions of women of all ages compulsively avoid such basic precautions? Ignorance about risks. Dread of finding an ominous lump. Delusions of invulnerability. Certainty that the discovery of a suspect nodule automatically spells premature death. Whatever the explanation, this dodging of responsibility comes under the heading of deeply ingrained health habits. Bad habits.

A 1992 study of 217 patients at the Strang Cancer Prevention Center in New York City found that the more anxiety women at high risk of breast cancer feel about developing the disease, the less likely they are to perform breast self-examinations and go for physician breast checkups. All the women in the study had a significant family history of breast cancer. Each patient had at least one "first-degree" relative (mother, sister, or daughter) who had contracted the disease. These women were two to three times more likely to develop breast cancer than those without such a family background.

A questionnaire given to participants in the study revealed that, despite this inherent hazard, only 69 percent of the women went for regular clinical breast exams. The other 31 percent delayed such follow-up visits for between nine months and two years. The survey also showed that only 40 percent of the women performed monthly breast self-examination, while 50 percent checked themselves only sporadically and 10 percent never did. Delusion and distress abounded in the women studied. The study found that 24 percent of the high-risk women believed they had little or no chance of developing breast cancer—but that another 27 percent were disturbed enough about the prospect of the disease to seek psychological counseling.

Mammograms, low-dose X-rays revealing the interior structure of the breast, can detect abnormal growths when they are smallest and most treatable, and can discover these lesions or densities, as they are called, as much as two to four years before they can even be felt by hand. According to the Federal Centers for Disease Control, mammography can prevent almost one in five deaths from breast cancer. Regular mammography screening that leads to early treatment for breast cancer can add one to 10 years to the life expectancy of a woman. From a broader perspective, mammography has raised the five-year survival rate for early breast cancer from 78 percent a few decades ago to 90 percent today.

Screening mammograms are generally recommended for women at least once by age 40, then either annually or once every two years from 40 to 49, depending on medical history, then every year for women 50 and over. Women with a family history of breast cancer are usually advised to get X-rays more often. As for monthly breast self-examination, it should be a routine health habit for women 20 and older. And clinical physical examination of the breast by a physician is recommended every three years for women 20 to 40.

Most breast lumps do not indicate cancer, but all suspect lumps should be biopsied for definitive diagnosis. The most common treatments include lumpectomy, the removal of a tumor and surrounding tissue, and mastectomy, the removal of a breast.

New, improved techniques make possible breast reconstruction after mastectomy.

The prognosis for survival of the disease has steadily improved. Among women under age 50 treated for breast cancer, nearly 80 percent live five years and about 60 percent live 10. For women older than 50, the numbers are similar: a five-year survival rate of about 75 percent and a 10-year rate of about 60 percent. All in all, the five-year survival rate for localized breast cancer has risen from 78 percent in the 1940s to 92 percent today. Ten years ago, only 3 percent of breast cancers were detected before they invaded adjacent normal tissue. Today, some studies show that the figure is 20 percent to 30 percent.

On the other hand, the U.S. government spends only one dollar on cancer-prevention research for every three dollars spent on cancer-treatment research. Some cancer experts increasingly advocate reversing that ratio. Breast cancer makes up more than 15 percent of all cancer cases, yet the disease accounts for only 5 percent of the $1.6 billion National Cancer Institute budget.

❧ ❧ ❧

"Okay, what are my options?" Barbara asked Sherman on hearing the diagnosis.

"You can have either a lumpectomy or a mastectomy."

"If I have a lumpectomy, what are the chances the cancer will come back?"

"Both approaches have proven to be about equally effective. You can have a lumpectomy followed by 26 days of radiation. Or you can have a mastectomy followed by six months of chemotherapy."

Barbara decided immediately on a mastectomy. She wanted all traces of breast tissue eliminated. If she were to err in this decision, it would be on the side of caution.

She asked Sherman, "Can you do reconstructive surgery on my left breast in the same operation as the mastectomy?"

He said, "Yes, you can have an implant put in."

But, she remembered thinking, My breasts will look different from each other. She also worried about her right breast developing a mirror tumor.

She said, "Well, if I have a mastectomy and reconstructive surgery only on my left breast, I'll probably feel slightly deformed. Can you do both breasts at the same time?"

"Yes," Sherman said, "but go home, think about it. Talk to a couple of plastic surgeons. You have a couple of weeks to decide."

"It was really as cut and dried as that," Norman recollected. "He told me I had breast cancer and I asked him what my options were. It was very businesslike, not emotional at all. I never got upset or cried. What would I have had to cry about? It could've meant I was going to die. But Sherman never led me to feel that I would. Something was wrong and we had to decide how to take care of it."

But it was not quite that easy. The day she had the biopsy, she went back to her office in midtown Manhattan. Sherman called her at work and said, "The pathologist just confirmed it—it's breast cancer."

She got into a cab to ride to Grand Central Terminal for the train ride home to Greenwich and thought, This is scary. Breast cancer can kill you. This is probably going to kill me.

"But that was my only bad moment—during that five-minute ride from my office to the station," she said. Then she remembered how Parke had dealt with his own difficulties. She thought, What can I do about it? We all have to die. I believe in God. I believe that we each have a certain time on this earth and can control only so much.

Barbara called her daughter Kathleen with the news. "I remember feeling in the pit of my stomach that this was unreal because I could never imagine anything happening to my mother," Kathleen recalled. "To be forced to think she was mortal was beyond the realm of my imagination. I was terribly distraught. Devastated. But I wanted to prevent my mother from getting upset. So I said, 'Okay, you'll be fine.'"

Worried, Kathleen came home from college to visit the plastic surgeons with her mother. After one discussion with a physician, Barbara walked out of his office and her daughter asked, "What are you thinking, Mom?"

"I have a feeling I'm not going to have any problem," Barbara said. "I think it's going to be all right. I just have this feeling. I have no idea why."

Kathy Salvo, too, remembers hearing the news from her friend. "I was really upset," she recalled. "I think it threw me more than her. I had just seen my cousin—a 21-year-old all-American lacrosse player—go through leukemia and die. I felt more frightened than she seemed. She was very calm and took it all in stride and said, 'Well, let's just see what happens.'"

What happened, in short, was this: On the morning of December 13, 1988, nearly two years after she had detected her lump, Barbara entered Stamford Hospital for bilateral mastectomies.

All of the tissue in both her breasts was removed, and she stayed in the hospital for five days to recover. "I left the hospital with these nice round little breasts," she said afterward. "No sagging to worry about. And I remember sitting there in the hospital, all bandaged up, and saying to myself, 'Hey, this isn't so bad.'"

About three days after surgery, Victor Grann, a Stamford oncologist, entered her hospital room and told her he had good news. Her tests showed that she was node-negative—meaning no cancer cells had spread to her lymph nodes. Barbara turned to Kathleen and said, "That's nice."

The morning after Barbara arrived home from the hospital, she walked her two dogs. Then she and Kathleen went out for lunch in Greenwich. In a few weeks, Barbara would go to Dr. Grann, to begin chemotherapy. All she knew, though, was that she wanted above all to get back into training. Back into the pool. Back on the bicycle. Back on course.

❧ ❧ ❧

"My father was a builder," Norman said. "A builder of homes. He had no particular training for it. As a young girl, I would go to building sites with him and carry lumber and watch him and the carpenters building houses. If a beam was out of line or a foundation seemed unstable, they would say, 'Listen, that's not working. Let's try this, or let's try that.'

"Years later, when I was about 22, my first husband and I bought a 200-year-old house in Stamford. It was pretty rustic, with a coal furnace in the basement, and it needed a lot of repairs. I was amazed at what I had learned from my father. Amazed at everything I could do with the house. Putting in lights. Installing wall sockets. Making connection boxes. Plastering walls. Putting down cement floors.

"So I was able to fix stuff, to solve problems. And maybe that's why I wanted to be a lawyer. Because that's essentially what I do in my job as a corporate lawyer: repairs. All day long, clients and colleagues bring me legal problems. Acquisitions. Divestitures. Litigation. Whatever. And they say, 'What are we going to do about this situation?' And I'll remember those carpenters who built homes with my father. I'll say, 'Let's try this, or let's try that.'"

❧ ❧ ❧

As Barbara sat in the waiting room on her first visit to Dr. Grann, she picked up a booklet titled *The Side Effects Of Chemotherapy*. By waiting-room standards, the booklet was hardly a diverting "read." Barbara scanned through the pages until she came across an especially memorable passage. It said that chemo might corrode the gums so much that a patient, in the interest of hygienic delicacy, would have to brush her teeth with a Q-Tip. Barbara thought that sounded pathetic, and her stomach gurgled. Just from reading a booklet. What, she wondered, might happen to her during treatment itself? One January afternoon, after she left her office for the day, Barbara found out: she had her first chemotherapy injection. She asked the nurse on duty with Dr. Grann that day the question foremost on her mind: "Do you think I'll be all right if I go for a swim right afterwards?"

The nurse said, "Well, I'm not sure I'd recommend that."

Norman asked, "Well, what would happen if I tried? Am I going to throw up in the car leaving here? Will I pass out?" The nurse said, "Tell you what. I'll give you some pills for nausea. And when you swim, just be cautious, take it very easy. I guess it'll be okay."

Norman drove directly to her swim club. She climbed into the pool and swam for about a half an hour and took it easy, just as the nurse had advised, and felt fine.

Her life, even given the logistical impediments of chemotherapy, assumed a new rhythm by the end of January. Once a week, in the late afternoon, she went to Dr. Grann for injections. She stayed on the medication, consisting of pills three times a day, for two weeks. Then she abstained from the drugs for 14 days. It would amount to a 28-day cycle of going on and off the medicine, repeated for six sequences, for a total of six months. "Her life hardly changed," said her daughter. "The chemo was hardly a blip on the screen."

Barbara and Kathy Salvo settled on a strategy: immediately after taking the drugs, Barbara would exercise as much as she could stand to water down the potential side effects. This program aimed a pre-emptive strike at the toxic chemo. She would go home from a visit with Dr. Grann and, within two hours, begin to run five miles, or zoom off on her bicycle, or swim laps at the pool club. She started slowly, then pushed harder. Often she teamed up with Kathy. They plotted a 13-mile course in Greenwich that swung around a yacht club and cut through a park.

"Barbara had a lot of faith in her physical strength," Kathy recalled. "She definitely believes that the body is what you make of it through exercise and diet. She felt that she had to stimulate her body to fight against whatever it is that might make it feel bad. She saw the chemo as another form of triathlon, and her fitness gave her great confidence about getting through it."

Barbara suffered only occasionally from nausea due to chemo. Sometimes her daughter would call her to ask, "How're you doing, Mom?"

And though Barbara would feel a little squeamish, she would say, "Oh, let's not talk about it right now."

Such stoicism was a matter of principle for Barbara. "I would never say I felt sick," Barbara recalled. "Just saying the words, I would feel ill. So I would never come out and say it. I'm the sort of person who sometimes denies that a problem exists. Or I never think about a problem. I just block it out.

"But even when I did feel nauseated, I went out and ran or swam or biked as hard and as fast as I could, and the queasiness immediately went away. My idea was that I would quickly sweat all the bad stuff from the drugs out of my system. That was my concept anyway: to sweat all the toxic stuff from my body. I really felt I could do that. I made myself sweat an awful lot—that was how I handled chemotherapy. I had no control over my breast cancer, but I did have control over the type of life I was going to lead."

If ever Barbara felt a twinge of an impulse to skip or soft-pedal a workout—as happened, though infrequently—Kathy injected her with a dose of motivation. One day, Kathy called Barbara to suggest a run together. But Barbara felt sick, and said, "Oh, I feel a little yucky today."

Kathy said, "Well, let's drive to this race course I know in Westchester—it's about four miles long—and the running will make you feel better."

"No, not that course," Barbara said. "It's too hilly. It starts with a mile straight uphill."

"We're going; we're leaving now," Kathy said, and they went.

As soon as they pulled up at the track, rain started pouring down, spattering the windshield. Barbara said to Kathy, "Oh, good, it's raining. Let's call it off."

Kathy, still behind the steering wheel, shook her head in rebuttal. "Oh no," she said, "we're going to run. Come on, let's go."

So out of the car they went, directly into this cold, pelting rain, and started striding along. The rain came down in torrents, and within minutes the dirt track had softened into rivulets of mud. Barbara and Kathy, both sopping wet from hair to running shoes, slipped and skidded along through puddles. Kathy would bolt ahead a few yards and Barbara, her competitive fires sufficiently stoked, would run harder and catch up. A quarter-mile later, Kathy would surge in front again, as if teasing her partner, and again Barbara would pull even. Over and over, they played cat and mouse, tit for tat, until they completed the course.

"By the end of that run, I felt wonderful," Barbara said. "Totally perfect."

For Barbara, Kathy turned out to be as much a close friend as a training partner. "Kathy always wanted to include me in her plans," Barbara said. "She would invite me to her parties, even though I was twice her age. She would say, 'We're having a party after the bike ride today. You want to come?' And I would say, 'But Kathy, I'm twice your age. I can't come to your party.' And then I would go anyway, and that was my group therapy.

"She filled some of the void I had in my life, and that was very helpful to me. All through the chemo, she set my sights not on my health problems but on training for races. She gave me a very special kind of support and encouraged me to compete. During training, she would say, 'Oh, come on, you can do better than that.' She never let me get down. I've said to Kathy, 'Where would I be without you?' She kept me sane right after Parke died and then during chemo. His death was more traumatic for me than my breast cancer. Kathy and I never discussed his death. I never told her how I felt being without Parke. But then, I never had to."

❦ ❦ ❦

All through 1989 Barbara (and Kathy) prepared for the Bud Light Ironman Triathlon World Championships—the World Series, the Super Bowl, the big Kahuna of endurance contests. Barbara turned in for bed at 9:00 p.m. every night. She woke at 5:00 a.m. the next day to train before work. She started slowly, running and cycling four, five, six miles a day through January. Then she upped the ante. By late March, she was running 32 miles, cycling 75 miles and swimming 8,000 yards every week. She seldom missed a day. She hung a poster of triathlon champion Mark Allen near a doorway in her laundry room to drive her on.

To counter the effects of chemo during the first six months of 1989, she also posted a chart for her diet, divided into categories: Protein, Carbo, Complex carbo, Fat, and, of course, Junk. Every day she noted the food she consumed, from cans of Exceed and granola bars to fettuccine with tomatoes and meatballs, and ice cream and cookies. She kept track of breakfast, lunch, and dinner, every day. Whereas she had once eaten light lunches—yogurt and rice cakes, say—she now made a point of tucking away an ample midday meal, more along the lines of thick fillets of chicken and heaping bowls of salad and pasta to maintain her strength.

As Barbara approached her second cycle of chemo, she registered for several triathlons, the better to psyche herself for a return to the crucible of competition. "Once I signed up for a race, I was extra motivated to train through the chemo," she said. "For an Ironman, you have to train a year. So I ate a lot, drank plenty of fluids, exercised excessively, and went to bed early. Chemo was not going to stop me from competing in Hawaii."

Visits to Dr. Grann confirmed that probably nothing would. Tests showed that her red- and white-blood-cell counts had stayed stable through chemo, rather than dropping precipitously as is usual. Dr. Grann marveled at the high blood-cell levels. He had never seen anything like it before. "What are you doing?" he would ask his patient.

Barbara also kept at her demanding job as a corporate attorney. She was vice president, secretary and general counsel for WMS Industries Inc., a New York Stock Exchange firm in Manhattan that owns hotels and casinos and also designs and manufactures pinball machines. She practiced out of the General Motors Building overlooking Central Park, just a few blocks from where Kathy Salvo traded stocks for Paine Weber.

In her highly cerebral job, Barbara refreshed herself from the rigors of the physical. She dealt daily with law in all its intricate complexities. With her specialty in securities law, she ensured that her company complied with the tenets of the Securities and Exchange Commission. On any given day, she might also counsel a senior manager on licensures or labor relations, or attend a board meeting, or need to call on her grasp of stock options and debentures. Contracts, leases, financing—she ranged all across the board. "Being busy—both in my training and at my job—prevented me from dwelling on anything negative," she said. "I never felt tired."

The training, the partnership with Kathy, her own will to persevere—all began to pay off for Barbara. In May 1989, her fourth month of chemo, she competed in the Gulf Coast Triathlon, a half-Ironman triathlon, against the scorching backdrop of Panama City, Florida. She started the event with Kathy and her daughter Kathleen. Among women over 50 years old, Barbara chugged to a first-place finish, qualifying for the 1989 Bud Light Ironman. Kathy made the grade, too. Eight days later, Barbara entered the Columbia Mid-Atlantic Regional Championships, in Columbia, Maryland, and came in second in the 50-plus category. One morning two weeks after that, she downed her last chemo pill. She raised the pill in front of Kathy, as if it were a glass hoisted aloft for a toast, and said, "Here's to my last chemotherapy pill." The same day, she competed in the Oxford International Triathlon, a half-Ironman in Oxford, Maryland. Once again— despite blistering 105-degree heat—she crossed the finish line ahead of all other women in her age group.

Norman competed in four major triathlons during her chemo, winning her age group in two. Without intending to gloat, she sent her oncologist, Dr. Grann, a newspaper article about her Oxford victory. Dr. Grann photocopied the profile and proudly showed it to his other patients. He contemplated writing a case study of her rapid recovery from breast cancer to publish in a medical journal.

By June, with her chemotherapy over, Barbara was training with Kathy harder than ever. Each week they averaged about six miles of swimming, 200 miles of cycling and 50 miles of running. If they worked out individually, they played one-upmanship, just to pump the levers of adrenaline. "We would turn our solo workouts into a big contest," Norman said. One would call the other to find out who had logged more mileage that day. "How far did you bike today?" Barbara would ask. "Oh, about 70," Kathy would answer. "Well, I biked 75," Barbara would come back. And they would laugh.

Through 1989, more than 4,000 competitors vied for the privilege to compete in Hawaii in October, in the Bud Light Ironman Triathlon Championship, against the best of the best. One hundred of the U.S. competitors were drawn from a lottery pool of 1,800 candidates. But most of the other contestants had qualified for the event by winning in 21 designated races in the United States that year.

In the five weeks before the Ironman in Hawaii, Barbara tapered her training regimen. The day before the race itself, though, she actually rode her bike two miles, just to keep herself loose and frisky as she laid it all on the line, big-time.

Moments before the Ironman, Barbara and Kathy cried with joy. "Both of us had talked about doing this race for two years," Kathy said. "It was like, 'Wow, we're finally here.' If felt like we had made it to the Olympics."

So it was that on October 14, 1989, Barbara Norman swam through the warm, clear waters of Kailua Bay, and pedaled her bicycle past the spooky lava flats with a shoehorn wedged in the back of her shoe, and trudged along in the cool dusk until she came across the finish line, gasping and smiling, third in her age group, and completed a personal odyssey far more profound than any single triathlon.

❦ ❦ ❦

In 1989 and 1990, *Triathlon Today* magazine named Barbara to its 50 to 54 all-American teams. In 1990 she notched age-group victories in six triathlons, including the Bay States Triathlon in the New England Series and the El Gran Trialo Bud Light Triathlon in Puerto Rico (Kathy Salvo came in second in the 25 to 29 age group). Norman concluded the season finishing first among the 50- to 54-year-olds at the U.S. Biathlon Federation National Championship in Central Park, New York. She even attracted a sponsor, Aerodynamics, a line of fitness apparel, the only 50-plus athlete so chosen. In 1991, *New England Runner* selected her the Senior Woman Triathlete of the Year. And in the summer of 1992, she posted a first-place finish in her age group at the Montauk Triathlon, where she had received her baptism of sweat as an endurance athlete nearly a decade earlier.

Barbara has raced in more than 40 triathlons. She has won many trophies but has never displayed these statuettes and plaques and certificates either in her home or office. She has no wish to tell others of her guts and stamina or to remind herself. When she recently moved from Greenwich to Chicago, she jettisoned most of these spoils. The award she most treasures is her survival. "Now I have a clean bill of health," she said. "Because my tumor was small, lymph nodes turned up negative and I had extensive chemo. My chances of recurrent breast cancer are less than 1 percent.

"As far as being a triathlete is concerned, I'm just an average person who has put time into three different disciplines," she said. "It's a matter of experience and practice and training and consistency. You have to know how to pace yourself and develop stamina and keep to your schedule. Anyone can do it, though, because almost anyone can run and swim and ride a bike. And if you do it long enough and well enough, you're bound to get better.

"All those early years I always thought that just finishing a race made me a winner. I felt that every time I competed, I won. Generally I would do my best, and if someone passed me, I would try to catch up. If I felt sick and I was pushing as hard as I could, then I would leave it alone.

"But in the last few years, especially since the Ironman, I've thought once in a while that maybe it's good to shoot for a win.

In some races, I've gotten into the spirit of trying to beat someone. Kathy has influenced me, made me think more about beating people. One triathlon in 1988, the Texas Hill Country Triathlon, was a sort of turning point. I had won the previous year and felt I had to defend my title. But coming out of the water from the swim, I was about 10 minutes behind the field. I saw a lady on the bike ahead of me and knew she was in my age group. I waited until we reached a big hill and, while she turned to look to the right, I zipped by her on the left. I had blisters on my feet and just killed myself to stay ahead of her. My time was 28 minutes better than the year before. I'll tell you—when your feet are all blistered and you run hard anyway, that's when you feel like a real athlete."

To act, to accomplish—it's Barbara's strong suit. Obstacles exist not to be sidestepped but to be overcome. "If she has six chores to do after work, she'll do every one," says Kathy. "I've seen her make dinner, paint the kitchen, and knit a sweater for someone, all practically at the same time."

Visit her house in Montauk. Though Barbara hardly knows you, she is solicitous. She offers you a seat, a drink, a stint with a video game, the bathroom, a stroll on the beach, a sumptuous lunch, whatever pleases you. If the blustery wind whipping off the beach is chilling her guests, she invites everyone to bivouac in the graveled driveway, the gusts now blocked by the house. If a lunch of herbed sliced chicken, tomato-and-basil salad, tortellini, and muffins holds no appeal for an eight-year-old guest, she unhesitatingly fixes him a classic peanut butter and jelly sandwich.

Here, too, one can bear witness to the partnership forged between Barbara Norman and Kathy Salvo, a bond that has extended well beyond the locker room. They team up even in the kitchen. Before a lunch for guests, they stand side by side at a counter, Barbara slicing tomatoes, Kathy placing freshly baked muffins in a basket. Together, they set the table and, later, put away the dishes. All with nary a word to each other. To this day, they follow the same routine, working out twice a day. But whether running or serving lunch, they remain in sync, linked by some rare telepathy, as close to one another as the closest of sisters.

Barbara seems averse, by and large, to looking inside herself with any depth or frequency. No sooner does she finish one chore than she segues to the next. Contemplation and introspection most assuredly do not win races or even, necessarily, combat disease. The day consists of tasks that, carried out and compiled, amount to a life lived to the fullest. It is this ethic of decisive action that has kept her in good stead as an attorney and an athlete. It is this philosophy, too, that has served her well as a cancer patient.

"I know I can do anything I put my mind to doing," said Barbara, looking back over challenges and travails. "I had worked as a secretary for a lawyer. Then I went back to college and, at age 37, went to law school to become a corporate lawyer. I've always felt that I can do it, whatever it is. All you have to do is believe. With my husband dying and my breast cancer, I never thought, 'Why does this stuff happen to me?' Something like this always happens. It's just part of life. But then you move on. Tell me I have breast cancer and we can try to fix it up. I did the same with the loss of my husband and my breast cancer as Parke had done about his condition: accepted it and, given the circumstances, did the best I could. Here's the problem. Now let's come up with a solution.

"That's just how I am—I've never dropped out of a race in my life."

Chapter 8

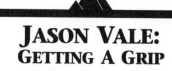

JASON VALE:
GETTING A GRIP

Lightning Bolt is praying.

After all, 24-year-old Jason Vale has to prep for his next arm-wrestling match. Vale is nicknamed Lightning Bolt because he pins opponents so fast. He takes down adversaries as if he's double-parked at a fire hydrant. On this warm Sunday night in June 1992, he squats near a platform stage with his head lowered, his hands clamped over his ears, and his eyes squeezed shut, the better to block out the clamor of the festival going on around him. He's getting what he calls "prayed-up."

More than a million people are thronging through Flushing Meadows Park to sample carnival rides, music, games of chance, and hot-off-the-grill food at the annual Queens Festival. But Lightning Bolt has come to grapple in the 15th Annual New York Pro Invitational Arm Wrestling Championship, sponsored by the New York Arm Wrestling Association. And to meet this challenge, the 5-foot, 11-inch, 182-pound Vale is praying hard. He rocks himself back and forth, a squint creasing the skin around his eyes, and tries to patch himself through on the switchboard to God.

The other two dozen competitors mill around behind the stage, where the trophies for each weight division are lined up on a makeshift shelf. These are rough customers here, truck drivers and construction workers, cops and former Marines. No Wall Street dilettantes need apply. Many arm wrestlers have arms like suspension-bridge cables, thick and striated from pumping weights. They run through private rituals designed either to psych themselves up or psych adversaries out, preferably both. They shadow-box or grandly flex the torso, and glare at likely opponents, or avoid eye contact.

Lightning Bolt, in blue jeans and a green T-shirt, goes through his own ceremony: he keeps praying. Even with more than a hundred hard-core arm-wrestling fans and curious passersby clustered shoulder to shoulder around him, he stays submerged in his trance. He moves his lips in silence, telling himself what he has to do. He calls for God to safeguard his soul so that, win or lose, he'll emerge from this tournament without feeling defeated where it counts—inside.

For the moment, he is oblivious to his surroundings. Onstage, competitors clash. The wrestlers sit at tables, directly opposite each other, and clutch each other with nutcracker grips. In the thick of a match, they wince and grimace, snarling and grunting through twisted lips. Jaws quiver from the effort, neck tendons pop out, cheeks puff out like those of adders. "Rip his arm off!" audience members scream.

Lightning Bolt is no newcomer here. He has won larger tournaments than this and comes in as a favorite. But this time he is competing in the 170-pound division, a heavier weight class for him. So he prays extra hard to come through with yet another victory in his usual no-nonsense, slam-bang, all-business, take-no-prisoners style. He's juicing himself up, hot-wiring his trip-hammer, bear-trap of a right arm with fresh volts of faith. His mother and father and brother and sister—all have witnessed this prepping ceremony of his before—know enough to stand back and leave him alone. Lightning Bolt powders his right hand with resin and takes the platform stage, to a chorus of whoops from family and friends. The Whitestone, New York resident has plowed through eight opponents to reach this stage in the event.

He's also overcome a long, bitter campaign against cancer. Only six years earlier, Jason had prayed for much higher stakes—his life. His back bears a scar from surgery and it's a doozy, a tire-tread imprint two feet long that curls under his left latissimus dorsi and swoops around beneath his shoulder blade, in a smiling crescent, past his spine.

Now he has surfaced as Lightning Bolt, and sits at a padded table facing Paul Walter of New Jersey. Walter rolls up the sleeve on his right arm, revealing a tattoo on his bicep. Hey, check me out, the move seems to say. Each contestant extends his right arm to clasp hands with the other guy and, with his left, grabs a six-inch-high post on the table for stability. They shift and squirm, jockeying in a tug-of-war for the right grip, an extra millimeter of turf, and finally unclasp. In arm wrestling, everything comes down to grip. More than a matter of comfort, grip gains an advantage, maintains equality, or gives away the marbles.

The referee, in black-and-white striped shirt, puts his hands on the tense lock between wrestlers. He pulls a thumb back over here, cocks a wrist an inch over there, sculpting the grip in a bid for balance. "You're up too high," he says. "Get down, now. Right there. Yeah, that's it. Now straighten up. Shoulders back. Okay, good. Let's do it, boys... Ready... Set... Go!"

Immediately Walter drives Jason back, like the hour hand of the clock tilting toward 1 p.m. Resin flakes off the hands of the wrestlers and flutters into the audience like specks of snow. "Rip his arm off!" a spectator yells. Walter keeps the pressure on and quickly gains ground, his wrist bending farther forward, lowering his adversary to within two inches of the table. Few wrestlers ever come back from such a disadvantage to win.

But now Lightning Bolt feels the spirit. "Pump it up, Jason!" his friends yell. "Pump it up!" He cranks his arm higher and higher, inch by inch, forcing Walter into retreat. The crowd cheers louder. "Get mean, Jason! Get mean!" Suddenly, they are dead even, both arms upright, back at Square One. But only for a moment, because now Vale switches on the auxiliary power. He turns his right shoulder toward Walter, adding torque, and presses him down toward the table. The audience is going nuts. Then Vale suddenly pins him and it's all over. Lightning Bolt has struck again, another prayer answered.

❦ ❦ ❦

In June 1986, six years earlier, Jason Vale ranked among the top handball players in Whitestone, Queens, a middle-class neighborhood consisting mostly of single-family residences in the second most populous borough of New York City. He had won handball tournaments and seemed likely to win more. A popular 18-year-old, handsome and athletic, he had just graduated from Holy Cross High School in Flushing, New York. He was playing handball every day as he prepared to leave for a job as a counselor in a summer camp. It was the best of times for him. Every day, in the schoolyard around the corner from his house, he slapped the hard rubber handball with an echoing "thwock" against a cement backdrop.

Then Vale started to cough. He coughed regularly and hard, short of breath. With each cough, he felt a throb in his left side, near his left lung and ribs, toward his back. Each day the pain grew more severe. He hurt worst at night when he lay down for sleep. Sometimes the pain seemed to emanate from directly under his heart, and Vale suspected he might suffer cardiac arrest in his sleep.

His parents took him to the emergency room at Flushing Hospital. A series of chest X-rays revealed, at the base of his left lung, a dark shadow on an otherwise white canvas. The attending physicians diagnosed pneumonia and prescribed intravenous antibiotics, but after a few days, the medications failed to improve his condition. Then the doctors thought he might have empyema, also an infection of the lungs. Nurses hooked him up to another IV solution and planned to administer more tests.

"No way," Vale said to his parents and the doctors in his whispery voice. "I'm not staying." The banquet for his high school graduation would be held in church that night, and he had no intention of missing it. "I've waited years for this," he said. "I'm going."

"Jason," his mother, Barbara, said. "You have to stay here in the hospital. It's for the best."

"There's nothing wrong with me," he insisted. "No way am I staying." And with that adamant refusal, he yanked the IV tube out of his forearm.

"What am I going to tell the doctors?" Barbara asked as he changed into his civilian clothes.

"You can tell the doctors whatever you want. Now take me home or I'll take a cab." Barbara declined to play accomplice in this act of defiance and her son walked straight out of the hospital. An hour later, doctors came to his room and found only Barbara.

"Where is he?" they wanted to know.

"What can I say?" his mother answered. "He's 18. He decided to leave."

"Well, something is not right. You better get him back."

Fat chance. Jason attended the graduation affair and went to camp, as planned. But again the pain in his side flared. He took more antibiotics, without benefit. He stopped eating and within six weeks lost 20 pounds. He sprawled in bed at camp, too agonized to move, and finally called his parents to pick him up and drive him home.

On August 10, he entered Booth Memorial Hospital in Flushing. Dr. Fouad Lajam, chief of thoracic surgery at the hospital, immediately ordered a CAT scan. Vale slid under the machine and lay still. Computerized axial tomography, or CAT, gives a cross-section view of the body with photographic "slices" one centimeter thick. By glimpsing otherwise invisible structures inside, a CAT scan can produce a more accurate look at an abnormality—its size, shape and location—than a conventional X-ray.

The scan revealed a sizable mass extending along the left chest wall, and Dr. Lajam told Mr. and Mrs. Vale that he suspected a cyst on the lung. Barbara Vale, a full-time homemaker with light freckles and short blond hair, and her husband Joe, a camera-store owner, listened quietly. Dr. Lajam explained that he needed to operate. He wanted to perform a surgical procedure known as a thoracotomy, primarily to draw excess fluid from the lung, and then explore to see whether anything else unseemly was going on inside Jason.

The boy underwent the operation the next day. Dr. Lajam sliced an opening from the scapulae, the two flat, triangular bones forming the shoulder blades, and carved deeply across the cavity of the chest to gain access to the lungs. Within a few minutes of getting inside, the surgeon discovered that the mass was no cyst. It was a tumor. The growth was about 15 centimeters wide and 25 centimeters long, roughly the size of a grapefruit, and fastened onto the chest wall. Gingerly, Dr. Lajam cut the tissue around the tumor and took it out. Because the growth was so large and deeply implanted, the delicate surgery lasted four hours.

Minutes later, Dr. Lajam went to the waiting room downstairs to tell the Vales. The physician favored candor over circumlocution. "We found a tumor," he said. The Vales gasped in unison. "And we removed it."

"Is it cancer?" Barbara asked.

"We're not sure," the doctor said. "We'll send it to the lab for the pathologists to examine and then we'll find out."

Three days later, Dr. Lajam received the biopsy report. "Unfortunately, it's malignant," he told the Vales. "But we still have to find out more."

Slowly, the Vales absorbed the verdict, and began to sob softly. Barbara thought, Now I have to tell Jason. Both parents went to his bed in the Intensive Care Unit. Jason lay pale and groggy, his eyelids drooping to half-mast, his mouth parched. Before the surgery, Jason had persuaded his parents to pledge full disclosure. "I want to know everything that's going on," he said. "Please, never hide anything from me or I'll never forgive you." The Vales had promised to inform him at every turn and now came time to make good on this vow.

"Jason," Barbara whispered. The boy turned his head on the pillow to look her in the eyes. "The doctors found that it's a tumor." She paused a few seconds to let the words sink in, before telling him the rest. "And it's malignant."

She will never forget his response to the news. "I was so worried about how he was going to take it," Barbara later recalled. "But Jason was so sweet. He was so strong. I'll never forget his first statement."

Without hesitating, Jason nodded and said, "It's okay... I'll be all right... God is going to heal me."

"Good," his mother said, and thought about it for a moment. "Yes... You're right."

❧ ❧ ❧

Barbara Vale taught Sunday school for 25 years. She also showed her own three children how to pray, starting with Jason and then moving on to his younger brother Jared and his sister Johanna. Before every meal, the family said "Grace" and every night she read her kids the Bible. The Vale family never missed Sunday or holiday services at the Free Gospel Church in Flushing.

From the beginning, Barbara set a proper example for her children. "I have a responsibility to God, to my children, and to myself," she explained. Jason readily invested himself in Christianity. "He always believed in prayer and faith," his mother said. "He would not only pray in church but also on his own." She would go to his room and see Jason in bed reading the Bible, or down on his knees, praying. Jason appreciated the teachings of the Bible enough by age 15 to memorize passages of scripture and compete on the Bible quiz team at the Free Gospel Church, where he ranked second in the district. Barbara would serve him dinner at the table, alone, and out of the corner of her eye she would notice him bow his head and, before he touched a morsel, begin to pray. "He always remembers," she said.

Jason channeled the same zeal toward athletics, the more competitive the better. In baseball, starting at age five, he played either shortstop or center field, both pivotal spots usually reserved for a team leader. Jason also enrolled in basketball and bowling leagues and engaged in pickup games of softball, touch football and street hockey. One Saturday morning Jason was playing center field, with his brother Jared stationed at shortstop, in a playoff softball game. With two outs, the batter lofted a blooper to short center. As Jason trotted forward, Jared back-pedaled, both of them calling, "I've got it! I've got it!" Neither heard the other, or much cared about this conflict of interest. Jason zeroed in first, caught the ball underhand, and accidentally slammed into Jared. The brothers crumpled to the outfield grass.

As they stood and brushed themselves off, Jason complained to Jared, "Hey, that was my ball." His voice growing higher and louder, he added, "The outfielder has the right to that ball. Anybody would know that." While the Vale boys came in from the field, Jason razzed Jared for trespassing on his turf. Barbara walked over to the bench to arbitrate between her sons. "That happens in the majors, too," she reminded Jason. "I saw an infielder and an outfielder collide on TV just the other day." But Jason, unappeased, kept backbiting about how Jared had almost blown the play.

"Jason was always very competitive," Barbara recalled. "He just tries very, very hard. He'd come home after a baseball game and mull over what he did wrong and how it happened, and call up his teammates and say, 'Come on, let's go to the batting cages and practice.' He was always more intense than the others. Sometimes he would get on people a little too much. He never let an argument go. With him, it could get like a Chinese water torture."

Later on, Vale switched to handball. He had fast hands and quick feet and pursued every ricochet. Soon he found that he preferred competing solo. You assumed all responsibility, depended only on yourself, received all credit and all blame. No collisions with teammates. In handball, he quickly learned the angles and the strategies, and could belt shots equally well with either hand. His confidence at the handball courts grew and he started to lay wages, $5 or $10 a game. He won a few games but lost money, mainly because he habitually challenged those whose prowess exceeded his. He would settle for nothing less than being the best in the neighborhood.

"Jason is competitive about everything, even chess," said his long-time neighborhood pal Johnny DiDonna, a student at Southampton University. "Loves to win, hates to lose. He was always very demanding of himself. In handball, he always wanted to play the top guys, just to keep getting better and better."

Vale befriended a guy named Flip, a 1979 world handball champion who acted as his mentor, and practiced every day; if you wanted real respect, you never stooped to shortcuts. He played hundreds of games against Flip, until the protégé had it all—the speed, the smarts—and could almost match the champ shot for shot. By high school graduation, Vale had become a first-rate New York City handball player.

Despite his Bible study and church visits and prayer, Vale was no angel, least of all in school. He wore sneakers, violating the dress code at St. Francis Prep, and ended up suspended. More than once he flung a tray of food in the cafeteria. He even climbed to the top of the school and scrawled graffiti. Once, he flirted with a young woman in the hallway, thinking her a student. She turned out to be a teacher and reported his impertinence to the principal. With religious regularity he got into such jams. For some reason, Vale always got caught. Though other kids would get away with boyish misdeeds far worse than his, he could never escape accountability. But because he believed in the Bible, he always knew when he had done wrong and admitted it.

Sometimes he crossed the line, though. Once, Vale and some friends got a master key for the high school storage room, and "borrowed" some band equipment (only to return it later, unsolicited). He also stayed out too late on school nights and came home to questions from his father about where he had gone. Joe was frequently frustrated at Jason's failures to return home by curfew and reveal his whereabouts.

Most serious of all, Jason developed a worrisome habit. He could always be counted on to get into nasty, knockdown fistfights.

❦ ❦ ❦

The tumor that Dr. Lajam removed from Jason Vale's left chest wall puzzled Susan Jormark, a pathologist at Booth Memorial. Dr. Jormark had never seen a growth quite like it, and had little idea what it might be, much less whether it might spread or how to treat it.

In the search for clues, Dr. Lajam ordered X-rays, CAT scans, sonograms, bone scans and magnetic resonance imaging for Vale, but the tests turned up nothing. All the physicians consulted on the case wondered why the growth gave no sign of metastasizing or invading any major organ. Sometimes a malignancy, once excised from the body, leaves in its wake a trace of microscopic cancer cells that require further treatment. Stumped, the Booth Memorial team sent the biopsy slides to Dr. Steven Hadju of Memorial Sloan-Kettering Cancer Center in Manhattan and Dr. G. Richard Dickerson of Massachusetts General Hospital in Boston, two of the leading pathologists in the United States.

By early October, Dr. Jormark had formed a provisional diagnosis. But rather than share her speculations with the Vales, she waited for the consensus from her colleagues at other institutions. As it turned out, her fellow pathologists at Memorial and Massachusetts General concurred with her suspicions. Vale had an exceedingly rare form of cancer. The growth was characterized, variously, as a small-cell sarcoma, a neuroepithelioma, and a perimative neuroectodermal malignancy. The bottom line is that it was an Askin tumor, named after Dr. Frederic B. Askin, the physician who had first detected it.

"We'll take it step by step," Dr. Lajam told Barbara. Booth Memorial at this point could do nothing else for Jason Vale. Dr. Lajam referred him to Dr. Peter Sordillo, an oncologist at Memorial

Sloan-Kettering who was one of the few specialists ever to treat an Askin tumor.

A letter dated October 6 bluntly spelled out the options facing Vale. Dr. John T. Fazekas, director of radiation therapy at Booth, sent the two-page correspondence to Drs. Lajam, Sordillo and Sidney Rabinowitz, the Vales' long time family physician. "The patient has recovered well and I believe there are plans for radiation therapy and chemotherapy," Dr. Fazekas wrote. "Physical exam reveals a pleasant and very healthy-appearing lad who looks his stated age of 18 and is in no apparent distress, totally recovered from his recent thoracotomy. His incision is beautifully healed and the lung exam is normal."

So far so good. But then the letter took a grim turn. The radiologist, in researching Askin tumors, had come across several articles on the rare malignancy, including a textbook chapter authored by Dr. Hadju of Memorial. The first research paper on Askin tumors appeared in 1979 in the journal *Cancer* and cited 20 cases. In the very last sentence of the letter, Dr. Fazekas wrote that each case culminated in "a uniform poor outcome and with essentially 100 percent mortality." By this circumspect jargon, Dr. Fazekas tried to convey a simple, undeniable fact: an Askin tumor is invariably considered fatal.

❦ ❦ ❦

If Jason Vale had a singular specialty as a boy, it had to be his talent for getting into fights. He had fights in elementary school, fights in junior high school, and fights in high school. He routinely came home with a bloody lip or a bruised jaw. He once had a front tooth knocked out. Twice had his nose broken. He seemed to have a confrontational, combative attitude that led to brawls wherever he went.

Barbara often heard about his aggression from teachers, friends and neighbors. "People would run up to our house screaming, 'Hurry up, Barbara! Jason's in a fight again!'" his mother recalled. "Or I would hear yelling and run outside the house and see an altercation with Jason in the middle of it. He would come home all beat up and want to go back. He told me that you had to face the other kid right away because otherwise you became afraid. So he would go right back out there. He was a fighter, plain and simple."

As his buddy Johnny DiDonna remembered, "When we were kids, Jason probably fought everyone on the block. I remember that he and I fought, too; we were angry about something, but I forget what. Anyway, every summer Jason would go away to camp and our block would get so quiet. Nobody would be fighting, and we realized it was because he was someplace else."

In fighting, rather than randomly lashing out, Vale followed a strict protocol. A would-be opponent had to fit certain criteria: be bigger than he; challenge him to fight, even if without words; and/or try to push around him or a friend of his. Vale always fought clean—no knees to the groin or gouging of eyeballs—and he never, ever, bullied anyone. And finally, as a matter of inviolate principle, he would throw the first punch. Always. "Some big kid around here would push you around, scream in your face, whatever, and it would look like he's about to give you a good shot," he explained. "You just anticipated his punch and delivered yours first."

"My father taught him always to strike first," said Joyce Vedral, his aunt, an author of self-help books and a former English professor. "That's his fighting philosophy." Sometimes Vale would dispatch the big right hand and knock a troublemaker out cold, the first punch also being the last. "I know how his face would look," DiDonna said. "Jason would get worked up to a point where there was no turning back. In his face I could always see it coming. Suddenly: boom!"

When Vale was about 15, Frankie Santos, who was taller and heavier than he, beat up his own friends with impunity. One night, Vale took offense at this rude practice. "Hey, Frankie," Vale screamed at him. "You always beat up your friends. What's your prob?"

"Shut up, pal," Frankie parried.

Vale, 30 pounds lighter and several inches shorter, waltzed over to Frankie and commenced screaming in his face. Frankie turned red. Witnesses swear he was about to unload some serious firepower on the upstart. Just then, Vale popped him square in the jaw, a pile-driver thrust that drove him to the pavement. This was a big event in Whitestone because until then, neither had ever lost a fight. They grappled on the ground, flailing away, gasping and grunting. Finally, Frankie stood, bruised and bloodied, and backed off, holding his palms aloft in a signal of surrender. Thanks to Vale, he never again picked on his friends.

"If Jason had gone into boxing, he would have become a champion," said his Aunt Joyce. "He has the strength and the guts and an incredible will. He's so strong it's scary. And he has a certain anger boiling inside him. His mother and his grandmother and I were always afraid that someday he would kill somebody.

He put more than one person in the hospital, just from one punch. I remember Jason once followed a drug dealer to a housing project in the middle of nowhere and punched him out with one shot. He ended up being unconscious for several days."

Barbara, neither proud nor ashamed, took a neutral stance on his penchant for fisticuffs. In mixing it up, she contended, he was simply taking care of business. "According to everyone I talked with," she said, "the fights never seemed to be his fault, and I believed that. Even in school, the principal would say Jason never seemed to provoke the fights. He was never disrespectful, never rude, never used foul language. His teachers always said he just had a lot of aggression that had to be channeled in the right direction.

"We had bullies around here who would take away your handball and kick you off the courts," Barbara continued. "I remember this one guy, Mike Rivera, who was about 17, and he always pushed around Jason, who was then about 14. I once warned Mike. 'You wait,' I said. 'In a few years Jason will be bigger and you'll have to cool it.' And one day about two years later, Jason had had enough. He must have done some number on Mike because the kid came here crying and said, 'Look what Jason did to me.' He had a gash in his mouth, and I got a cold cloth and wiped away the blood. He went to the hospital and needed 14 stitches. But he said he had no hospitalization insurance. And you know what? Jason let him borrow his Blue Cross card.

"I never did get to the bottom of all those fights," Barbara said. "I talked with Jason about it until I was blue in the face. I would ask him to reason with people rather than settle everything with his hands. He's very powerful and I was worried that he would really hurt someone with that right arm of his. As Jason got older, my husband would say to him, 'You better be careful. Your punches are getting lethal. One day you'll hit someone and by accident he'll crack his head on the concrete and die and you'll go to jail.'"

Jason felt lousy about his easy intimacy with violence. "I'm not going to do it again," he would tell his mother. "I'm really going to try to cut it out."

"It's not like he tried to justify the fights to me," Barbara said. "He felt bad."

Hard-pressed to understand his actions, Jason explained, "The fighting had to be done. I'm not saying it was right or wrong. But some fights just had to happen."

Maybe it was just as well. Whatever his motivation, Vale would later draw deeply on this readiness for battle. It would come in handy when he faced a deadly bully named cancer.

❦ ❦ ❦

The day Vale came home from the hospital, he felt pretty full of himself, certain he had the disease licked. He decided to show off for his friends, despite the staples still embedded in his back from the thoracotomy. He bent over, pressed his palms down on the driveway alongside his house and sprang into a handstand. He maintained this upside-down position, with his arms quivering from the strain, for a few long seconds. See? the gesture declared. See what I can do? I'm as good as new. No cancer is going to push me around.

The next day Jason found out otherwise. He invited his brother Jared to play some handball. Although Jared was athletic in his own right, Jason was bigger, stronger, and faster, and had always prevailed in such contests. The score stayed close from the start, seesawing as Jared edged ahead and Jason inched back. But ultimately, Jason lost to his kid brother for the first time. "I was very upset about that," Jason remembered. It dawned on Jason that if you go through an eight-hour operation to take out a grapefruit-sized tumor from your chest, you just might wind up the lesser for it on the handball courts.

Yet his newfound humility was short-lived. He craved the rough-and-tumble contact of street hockey; he wanted to roller skate along at high speed and whack at the puck with his stick and slam into somebody. He felt compelled to pit himself against an opposing force, if only to measure himself. For him nothing could articulate better than competition what he had inside himself.

Dr. Lajam warned Vale to avoid contact sports. The intensive surgery had left his midsection fragile and vulnerable, and street hockey might subject him to body blows of concussive force, undermining his recovery. Vale begged the physician for permission to play. "Please," he pleaded. "I'll be careful." And the doctor said, "Well, maybe it'll be okay if you get a special brace."

Vale visited a local sports equipment shop and bought such a brace. The padded, customized brace fit tight around his waist, like some kind of corset, and hampered his movements. Playing street hockey in the protective device, he felt stiff and straight-backed, slow to swivel on his skates. But at least the brace shielded his ribs from injury. And with Vale back in action, his team voted him to be its captain, and then won more often than not.

"That's how determined Jason was to get back to normal in a hurry," his mother recalled. "He was going to play hockey, no matter what. This upset me more than his fights used to. I was afraid he would hurt himself skating around in the streets. I think he wanted to prove something—to himself and the rest of us. Prove that he was not going to lie back, that he still had the right stuff. He was going to do what he always did: take everything into his own hands."

Meanwhile, Barbara kept the letter from Dr. Fazekas tucked in her pocketbook. She frequently pulled it out to read again, but the words about poor outcome and 100 percent mortality never changed. She grasped the jargon all too well. The other patients had died. Only one interpretation seemed possible. Jason would die, too.

Barbara wanted to conceal the letter from him, but she remembered her promise. If she neglected to tell him everything that was going on, he had threatened never to forgive her. Finally, she showed Jason the letter. Fazekas, he saw, regarded him as all but officially terminal. But even with this prognosis, the 18-year-old kept himself in check. He repeated to his mother what he had said in the hospital on first hearing about his cancer. "It's okay... I'll be all right... God is going to heal me," he said.

Now the Vales had to come to terms with the issue of treatment. Dr. Sordillo of Memorial reviewed the case and referred Jason to Dr. Edward J. Beattie, an internationally eminent thoracic surgeon, and Dr. Noel Raskin, also a thoracic surgeon, both of whom agreed that Dr. Lajam had scraped away the tumor, leaving no hint of lingering cancer. Accordingly, they called for the standard next step—radiation and chemotherapy—to prevent the tumor from growing back. Dr. Raskin wrote a letter to Sordillo saying, "As this tumor is apparently quite aggressive, I think careful follow-up is certainly needed."

I want to find out for myself, Jason thought. So one fall morning, he and his father Joe drove over the Whitestone Bridge, along the Cross-Bronx Expressway, down the East Side Drive into Manhattan, and headed for the library at the New York Academy of Medicine over in Morningside Heights. With Joe looking on, Jason flipped through the card catalogue. Askin tumor, Jason said to himself. Where is Askin tumor? References and citations about the disease are about as rare as the condition itself. Jason rifled through the voluminous records, Joe marveling at his initiative and industry. Why should I listen to the doctors? Jason asked himself. I want to know the real deal for myself. Within an hour he had discovered what he needed to know.

It was true, just as the Fazekas letter said: All of the patients who contracted Askin tumor died from it. In every case documented, the malignancy had spread quickly and killed the patients, always within a year. But wait a minute now. Look here. This was a fact no doctor had mentioned to him. All the Askin tumor patients covered in the medical literature had gone through radiation and chemotherapy, the same treatment recommended for him. Result: the tumor would fade away, seemingly obliterated, only to resurrect itself within a month or two. The therapy made no difference. The patients died anyway.

Why bother? Vale thought. If the chemo and radiation failed with others, why would they work on me? Maybe the doctors just killed those patients faster. Maybe treatment does more harm than good. Maybe, he thought, he should just pray—and by praying, get in the first punch.

So Vale decided against therapy, just flat-out refused to go through with it. No radiation would beam down onto his chest; no chemo would seep into his system, either. Not if he had anything to say about it. "I believed I could take care of myself," he said. "Cancer was just something else in my life I would have to fight."

His physicians pressured Vale for the next six months to accept treatment. Dr. Rabinowitz, his family physician, urged him to get therapy, and so did the surgeons Dr. Lajam and Dr. Raskin and the radiologist Dr. Fazekas. Oncologist Dr. Sordillo was so concerned that in March, 1987, he wrote Vale a certified letter "to emphasize again to you how strongly I feel that you not continue to delay treatment for your condition." Sordillo went on, "As you know, I have felt strongly since you first came to see me that you should be on chemotherapy to try to prevent your tumor from coming back... Dr. Raskin and I have spoken numerous times about you and we spoke again today... Please do not delay any further in allowing us to do this."

Barbara had plenty of time to think through this controversy. The upshot was that she put limited stock in what the doctors said. Go ahead, say your piece, she thought. I'm sure you went to a terrific medical school and I appreciate the letter. But what you should understand here is that this is Jason Vale we're talking about and he's my son. He's another story altogether. So let's not get bogged down in facts.

Jason believed he could recover on his own, and his faith was catching. "I believed every case was different and I knew Jason was a fighter," Barbara explained. "He took the initiative and I felt he was making rational decisions. He was not going to abandon all medical help. But we just decided he would refuse the treatment and we would take it from there. Prayer can change everything, and now we would pray together."

Jason prayed that, in declining treatment, he had decided for the best. "That whole first year of cancer, I felt overwhelmed by my faith in God and the hope He gave me," he recalled. "God just planted faith in my heart and mind and I went ahead without any chemo or radiation. I had faith that He was going to take care of me and work it out somehow and I was going to keep on going. I never felt defeated inside and I never thought about dying. The idea that I was going to die never even came into my head."

The months passed, and Jason returned to handball. He swore to his mother, in her moments of doubt, that he would be all right, and after he turned 19, he seemed to be back to normal, warrior spirit and all. One day a huge teenager named Tenny, who weighed nearly 400 pounds, rode by the handball courts on a motorcycle with his girlfriend clutching his torso. Jason waved an innocent hello to the girl and Tenny, taking exception to such hospitality, climbed off his bike and cursed at Jason. The recovering cancer patient was in no mood to fight and expressed his lack of evil intent in waving hello. Tenny grabbed his shirt and that's all he had to do. Jason landed a shot flush on his jaw and Tenny toppled like a redwood, out cold.

For more than a year now, Jason had skipped chemo and radiation without suffering adverse consequences. With his patented first-strike capability, he had rendered unconscious a motorcycle thug more than twice his size. Against all odds, the kid seemed to be in the clear.

❦ ❦ ❦

But not for long. In the fall of 1987, now enrolled as a freshman at Queens College, Vale felt the same pain as he had endured a year earlier, in exactly the same spot along his left side, the site where Dr. Lajam had discovered the Askin tumor. The pain was so bad it prevented him from sleeping on his back, but however much he tried to lie on his stomach and side, it kept him awake all night. Even to walk tormented him. The relentless pain upset his balance and he swayed from side to side as he climbed stairs, resorting to the railing for reassurance, stepping as if on hot coals.

The pain grew progressively worse and degenerated into agony. He wanted to chalk up the pain to handball, to twisting his torso too abruptly in swatting a shot and pulling a muscle or ligament.

But he saw no profit in trying to kid himself. Maybe bypassing treatment was a mistake after all. Maybe the tumor had recurred.

Dr. Rabinowitz prescribed Percocet, a narcotic, and recommended the standard dosage regimen of two pills every four hours. But even heavily medicated, the boy found little relief. Once the drug wore off, the pain came back. Day by day, as he built a tolerance to the chemicals, the pain returned sooner and sooner. And with each resurgence coming on the heels of a lull, the pain would feel harsher, more jagged and piercing.

Vale begged God to take away the pain, prayed for the pain to migrate out of his body and into the ether. It was a simple proposition. If the pain left, he could play handball and study for college. He could sit, stand, and walk without difficulty. He could sleep through the night. Granted a reprieve from the smoldering in his side and back, he could even envision a life without cancer.

"Jason was in such pain all the time," Barbara said. "It got to the point where he could not lay down in bed. He would sit in a chair all night because the pain was so bad. I'd fall into a fitful sleep and get up during the night because I knew he was still sitting there, unable to sleep. I was dying inside, seeing him in such constant pain. It hurt me so much."

Desperate for relief, Jason found unendurable the four-hour wait between drug doses and grew more and more impatient. One day he held off for only three hours before popping another pair of Percocet, if merely to walk or sleep comfortably for a spell. Then he shortened the delay to two hours, and finally to only one. Now, instead of downing two Percocet every four hours, he liberally medicated himself with six every three hours, more than thrice the recommended quantity. He went through a vial of 20 pills in half a day. And Dr. Rabinowitz had no intention of giving him a refill. So Jason forged prescriptions, a violation of federal law. To the figure "20" on the Rx vial, representing the number of pills, he added a zero. The unsuspecting local pharmacist then dispensed 200 Percocets. "I had to," Vale said, "because nobody would believe the pain."

Barbara believed it. She could see it for herself. But she worried he had gotten hooked. "We argued about his taking all the pain-killers," she said. "I would hide the pills and dole out only what I thought was necessary."

Sometimes Jason would lie in bed on his stomach and his mother would massage his back. She would rub the site from which the piercing pain emanated, the spot on the left side of his back, under the shoulder blade and around the ribs, the same location where the Askin tumor had swollen and the surgeons had done the thoracotomy. Barbara would press her fingers into his muscles to muffle the pain, and after an hour her knuckles and wrists ached. "Pray with me," Jason would say to her as she kneaded his back, and they would pray together. He put credence in the science and folklore that surrounded the laying on of hands. "Whenever my mother massaged my back," he recalled, "it was like magic. The pain would go away. I was so thankful that I wanted to cry."

❦ ❦ ❦

However much Jason wanted to depend on narcotics, massage, and prayer, his father now urged him to go in for a CAT scan. "We have a CAT scan scheduled in two days," Barbara said. "No," Joe replied. "Call *now*. He has to go in *now*." The Vales alerted Dr. Beattie. And on October 14, 1987, Jason hobbled into Beth Israel Medical Center in Manhattan, flanked by his parents, who held him upright and guided him into the emergency room.

Quickly, an orderly wheeled the boy into an X-ray suite. Dr. John M. Cosgrove, chief surgical resident, examined him first. "Jason was lying on a stretcher twisting around and grimacing in pain, yet still upbeat," Cosgrove recalled. "We shook hands and I could tell, just by his grip, that he was strong. He gave me such a tremendous squeeze."

Now Vale had to lie down straight and stay still for the CAT scan to pass over him. The doctors had to see inside his chest to find out whether the tumor had again cropped up. But the pain in his back prevented him from sufficiently uncoiling his body to lie flat. An anesthesiologist dosed him with Demerol, then morphine. The nurses then injected him in the spine with a contrast dye, for a clearer, more telling CAT scan image. As the machine hummed over him, photographing away, Jason drifted into a painless sleep.

The next day, a radiologist led Jason into a room to look at film of the results. There, on a brightly illuminated screen, the boy at last glimpsed the source of his pain. "My body had a new tumor," he said, "and I saw it for myself. Now I knew exactly what it looked like. It was a white spot where it was supposed to be dark, near my left lung. It looked like a big white cloud. Like a ghost."

The size of a fist, the chest-wall malignancy had grown on his left lung, close—perilously close—to his spinal cord. The Askin tumor, reprised, had begun to eat away at bone, compressing his spine. This growth represented a new danger: complete, permanent, irreversible paralysis of the legs. If allowed to spread over the next 48 hours, it threatened to render Jason paraplegic.

The surgeons would have to go in again, no later than the next day.

Dr. Beattie would supervise the second operation at Beth Israel, with Dr. Cosgrove at his side. This time, the doctors would perform a laminectomy; they would remove three ribs, a section of his left lung, and about three inches of his spine. That afternoon, the white-haired, grandfatherly Dr. Beattie swiftly pressed into service Drs. Cosgrove and Raskin, neurosurgeon Richard Bergland and the rest of the multi-disciplinary surgical team and diagrammed the details of the procedure on a blackboard. All the health-care professionals attending this briefing had a sense, given the rarity of the tumor, that this was an operation of some historical import.

That night, at the Free Gospel Church in Flushing, where the Vales had attended services for many a year, Pastor Marvin Boyce led a special service for Jason. With several hundred congregants listening, including family and friends, Boyce announced that Jason would undergo major surgery the next morning at nine. "Let's remember Jason Vale in our prayers," the pastor said. "He's in a lot of pain, but we believe God will heal him." Boyce recited passages of scripture to illustrate the restorative powers of the deity. The Pentacostal congregants knelt in the pews, heads bowed and hands clasped, and prayed for Jason. Some members of the flock shouted "God heal him!" Others sang "Hallelujah!" All the prayers came together, fusing into a single voice, a choral plea for mercy floating toward the heavens.

Jason remained in the Intensive Care Unit that night, closely monitored. If his condition worsened, Dr. Beattie would operate ad hoc. Every hour through the long evening, with paralysis still an imminent threat, the nurses approached Jason to make sure his legs still had feeling. They would tickle his foot and, reflexively, he would kick.

The next morning, Jason awoke and opened his Bible. He read in Romans 5 the following verse: "We also rejoice in our sufferings, because we know that suffering produces perseverance; perseverance, character; and character, hope." In these words, he found comfort. "In my heart I felt this peace," he said. "That was all I had to read to be happy." He took the Bible with him down to the operating room and pored over more passages. "God spoke to me on the operating table. It was like He was right there with me, speaking to me through the verses." As 9 a.m. neared, an orderly asked Jason to close the book. "Relax," a nurse told the orderly. "Let him read his Bible."

In the operating room, Team Vale—six surgeons, three anesthesiologists, and two nurses, all scrubbed and ready—gathered around Jason to exorcise this stigmata.

"Do whatever you have to do," Jason told Dr. Beattie.

Cosgrove felt butterflies swooping through his system. The doctor, himself age 29, only 11 years older than his patient, had played football at Harvard University and had quickly come to feel a special rapport with the young, athletic Vale. Likewise, Jason sensed a growing affinity with the 235-pound, crew-cut Cosgrove and his brisk, drill-sergeant manner. "Many people at the hospital thought Jason would not survive," the doctor recalled. "In the back of our minds, all the surgeons involved thought his lesion was lethal."

As Jason inhaled anesthetic through a tube in his throat, his eyelids drooped, his breathing deepened, and his head sagged to the side. He seemed to have sunk into unconsciousness.

Then he suddenly bolted upright on the operating table, eyes wide open. "Fooled you!" he taunted. For a moment, everyone stood flabbergasted, saying nothing. Then Team Vale exploded in laughter, Jason included. The comic prank, so exquisitely timed, defused the tension in the room. "At first, nobody could believe it," Cosgrove said. "Everyone thought Jason was out cold, but he was only a little groggy. The anesthesiologist rolled her eyes and laughed and said she had never seen a patient do that before. He fooled us, all right, but it was positive and upbeat. It put us in the mood to really rock and roll and get the tumor out. I think Jason was also trying to send us a signal: that he still had some control of the situation."

Finally, Jason went under, no kidding around now.

The surgeons cut through the scar tissue formed around the incisions made by Dr. Lajam in the thoracotomy at Booth Memorial 15 months earlier. With painstaking finesse, and in perfect synchrony, Drs. Beattie, Cosgrove, Raskin, and Bergland set about taking out pieces of Jason Vale, the better to clear a path to the fist-sized Askin tumor that again threatened to kill him. With the tumor now spreading in the spinal canal, any and all roadblocks had to come loose.

Out came three ribs from his left side, the surgeons also paring away the surrounding tissue. Out, too, came a section of his left lung, three thoracic vertebrae in his backbone, and the nerves connecting ribs to spine. Dr. Bergland operated directly on top of the spinal cord. Any false move, such as an errant severing of the cord, would mean lifelong paralysis. Only after clearing all roadblocks could Dr. Beattie reach in through the chest and snip away at the potentially fatal malignancy, until he had plucked it clean from the body and could hold it aloft in the sterile air where no harm could come from it.

Now, with the 18-year-old boy so rudely laid open, Dr. Beattie had to close the flaps of his chest. The only problem was that so much of the skin from his chest was gone. So the surgical team pieced together a synthetic mesh, much like a scaffolding, to seal the exposed cavity. Given the copious bleeding, the doctors transfused Jason with five units of blood, about a liter in all, one-third the amount available in the average human body. The laminectomy had lasted eight hours.

Moments later, Beattie came out of the operating room and told the Vales that Jason was fine, resting in stable condition. Barbara and Joe wanted to know whether the boy would walk. Too early to tell, the doctor answered. And what about the tumor? Probably all gone, Cosgrove said, but again, too early to tell.

The doctor took the Vales to the recovery room to see Jason. The boy remained woozy, unable to speak. "We're praying for you," Barbara said. She grazed her hand against his cheek and leaned over to hug him. Then Cosgrove took the opportunity to conduct a test on Jason. He flickered his fingers along his right foot to tickle the slumbering boy. If Jason moved his foot, the doctor explained, it meant no paralysis. Instantly, the foot twitched.

Only later would the parents find out that Joe, in his insistence on taking Jason in immediately for a CAT scan, had saved the day. Had the Vales waited another 24 hours to bring the boy in, Jason might have ended up paralyzed for life.

❦ ❦ ❦

The second surgery was not the end of his troubles but only the beginning. Jason would need at least two weeks in the hospital to get going on his recovery. The staff in the Intensive Care Unit at Beth Israel had to cast a vigilant eye on him. When he moved into a regular room on the third day, his parents bought him a TV and an electronic chess set to keep him occupied (read: out of trouble). On the fourth morning, Dr. Cosgrove visited Jason and his parents. "This young man will have to get treatment this time," he said. But Jason remained unconvinced, even now, that he should go through chemo and radiation.

The boy would collect no trophies as a model hospital patient.

He refused to eat, complaining the food was lousy, and went eight days without a shower. The doctors ordered him to stay in bed, but he got up by himself anyway. A few times he pretended, once upright, to stumble to his knees, a stunt somehow amusing to Jason but unnerving to the nurses. "He clowned around, trying to throw the nurses into a panic," Barbara recalled. "But nobody thought any of this was funny."

Nurses came into his room all day to carry out routine chores. They brought in his meals, drew blood, checked his blood pressure, changed the bed sheets, took out the garbage, cleaned the bathroom. If a nurse came into his room to give him a shot, Jason would ask, "What's in the needle?" Once, a nurse replied, "Don't worry about it." He said, "Well, I want to know what you're giving me and I want to know why." He hated being so closely watched, hated letting everyone do everything for him. After a week, he took a stand. He refused to let the nurses put on clean sheets. He pulled shut the curtain around his bed, the better to maintain a semblance of privacy, as if to enfold himself in a cocoon. He wanted to a hang a sign on the door to his room saying DO NOT DISTURB. "The nurses came in 30 times a day and it bothered me," Jason said. "I never got to sleep. Some days I shut my door so nobody would come in." Twice the hospital sent in a psychiatrist to visit him.

Jason ran a fever and went on intravenous antibiotics. He blamed the fever on the antibiotics and snatched the IV tube out of his forearm and let the medicine dribble into his urine bottle. A doctor, exasperated at these hi-jinks, called Barbara. "I'm taking myself off this case," he said. "If your son isn't going to listen to me, I'm not going to be responsible."

The doctors took Jason off Percocet, despite his continuing pain. "I would wake up in the middle of the night hurting so much," Jason said. "It was the worst." This sudden withdrawal from the narcotic left Jason thin-skinned and cranky. One day an intern went to his room and, unprovoked, sat on his bed and called him "truculent and cantankerous." Jason preferred to keep his bed to himself and resented this presumption. "Get off my bed or I'm going to punch you in the face," he threatened. Barbara, right there, blushed.

Startled, the intern said, "See? You're truculent and cantankerous." Jason looked at the intern and adrenaline surged through his system. He stopped feeling pain at that moment. Intoxicated with fury, he wanted to take a swing at the doctor.

The comment became a running joke between him and his mother. If Jason acted pigheaded or protested too much, Barbara would tease, "Jason, you're being truculent and cantankerous." By the same token, if Jason caught himself acting stubborn and temperamental, he would coyly ask, "Mom, tell the truth. Am I being truculent and cantankerous?"

Most of all, Jason hated the tubes. The surgeons had carved a gaping hole in his chest and plugged in two thin tubes to drain excess blood and fluids and to vacuum out air to prevent his diminished left lung from collapsing. The tubes bubbled all day from the suction, and relayed the accumulated discharges into a gurgling collection device that reminded Jason of an aquarium. "This is useless," Jason told the hospital staff. "Get these tubes out of me."

He just wanted to get out of there. Fed up with the indignities of hospital life, Jason wanted to detach himself from the fish tank and go home. He believed he could take better care of himself in his own house. So he plotted The Great Escape.

He called his friend Jo Marie Penna. "Listen," he said, "I could lay around like this at home and still get better. I'm leaving the hospital."

"Leaving?" Jo Marie said.

"Yeah."

"What do you mean leaving?"

"Walking out. I can't stand it here anymore. I want you to come in from Queens and drive me home."

Jo Marie, along with her friends Therese DeCarlo and Julie Shu, went to Beth Israel on the pretext of an ordinary visit to Jason. But when they arrived planning to take him home, the three young women noticed the tubes poking out of his chest. The tubes burbled and looped into a repository, like a portable septic tank, that Jason pulled alongside him as he walked.

"You're not leaving," Therese said. "I'm not driving you home."

"You *have* to drive me home," he said.

"No," she said. "I don't and I won't. Not with all those tubes sticking out of your chest."

"If you're not going to help me out," Jason said, "I'll leave on my own."

With that statement, his three friends left. Jason disconnected the tubes from the tank and coiled the ends dangling from his chest under his overcoat. He stepped outside his room and looked down the hall—left, then right—to check whether anyone who knew him was coming. He might encounter too many people in an elevator, so he took the stairs and walked down from the seventh floor to the lobby. He headed toward the front door, passing the security guard, and made it outside, his hospital gown peeking out below the hem of his coat. He felt so tired. For a moment, he just stood there out on Second Avenue near 17th Street in Manhattan, breathing in the open air. He went to a pay phone planning to call a cab.

Instead, he called his mother. Barbara answered on the second ring.
"Hi, Mom."

"Jason, I hear a lot of cars and trucks. Is your window open?"

"No, Ma, I'm downstairs in the street, at a phone booth. I'm not staying here anymore. You have to come get me or I'm going to take a cab."

"Jason!" she screamed.

"Ma, I'm not staying in the hospital for one more minute."

"What about the tubes?"

"Listen, that's nothing."

"Are you walking around with the tubes coming out of you?"

"I'll take the tubes out myself at home. I can do that without a doctor."

"Jason!" she screamed again. "Don't do this! You *can't* do this, for God's sake! You're going to injure yourself."

"But Ma…"

"… No, you listen to me very carefully. Nobody knows you're gone yet. Nothing will happen, no repercussions, if you quietly go back upstairs and sneak back into your bed. *Please!* If you honor your mother and father, if you have any fear of God, you will get back in that hospital!"

So much for The Great Escape. Jason said goodbye and hung up the phone. He went back into Beth Israel and rode the elevator to the seventh floor. He shrugged off his overcoat, climbed back into bed and called for a nurse. It seemed the tubes had come loose, he told her. Could she please fix them?

"All I know is, I was beside myself," Barbara recalled. "How was I going to make this kid listen? He gave everybody a very hard time: the doctors, the nurses, and me. Usually, when something traumatic happens, I just shift to a lower gear and become ultra-calm. I think, Okay, something has happened. Let's see what we can do about it. But this time I just lost it."

Drs. Cosgrove and Beattie later that day got wind of the incident. Beattie, incensed at this flouting of the rules, threatened to kick Jason out of Beth Israel. But Cosgrove, feeling protective, stepped in and told Beattie he would take care of the kid.

That son of a gun, Cosgrove thought. He actually disappeared from the hospital with tubes coming out of his chest. That's how much he wanted to get out of here. I'm going to go up there and kick his butt.

The young surgeon immediately paid Jason a little visit. "I was concerned about his cocky attitude," Cosgrove said. "I told him he'd better straighten out his act and that we're the bosses in the hospital. I told him he'd better do what we say if he wants to get better, and that if he pulled a foolish stunt like that again, it would just prolong his hospitalization. He promised it would never happen again. It was impossible to get mad at him. He'd gone through so much." Cosgrove later told Barbara that Jason, in pulling the tubes from the tank, had run a serious risk. If the tubes had popped out of his chest, his lung could have collapsed. Such an accident might have invited an infection. He could have died.

Cosgrove suspected that Jason would persist in his refusal to cooperate. The physician stopped in on him two or three times a day, not only to check him but also to lecture him. "I felt a special fondness for the kid because we were so close in age and both played sports," Cosgrove said. "I knew he would be a tough patient. But I'm tougher. I knew that if anyone could bring him around, I could."

❦ ❦ ❦

Jason finally relented on treatment and went in for emergency radiation therapy a few days before Thanksgiving. He lay on a table and let technicians mark his back with blue emblems designating the site of treatment. Then the radiologists fired high-energy ionizing radiation at the spot to kill any vestiges of cancer cells. The plan was to blast him with radiation for 30 straight days. Such treatment snaps the strands of DNA molecules inside these cells, preventing the cancer from growing and dividing. The first round of radiation rendered his mouth raw inside, so dry he became unable to swallow his own spit. But the treatment shrank the unidentified swelling in his back and Cosgrove put Jason on morphine and steroids to ease the pain and inflammation.

During the second such session, Jason thought, I should just walk out now. Walk out and never go back. Not for this.

No matter that he had come so close in the last year to paralysis and death.

Now Cosgrove arranged for the radiation department at Beth Israel to stay open on Thanksgiving just for him. Despite his appointment, Jason had a better idea: a sequel to The Great Escape. He called his cousins Eric and Cory Dash to drive him home to Whitestone for a surprise visit with his family on Thanksgiving. Here a major New York City hospital had kept open an entire department specially for him, at considerable expense. But Jason nonetheless put on a raincoat, ducked into a cab with his cousins and showed up, unexpected and unannounced, at the Vale residence. His parents and siblings were there, and so was Grandma, along with some aunts and uncles, all hovering over a buffet of turkey, stuffing, candied sweet potatoes and baked-cheese macaroni.

"He walked in the door during Thanksgiving dinner looking emaciated," recalled his Aunt Joyce. "I thought he was going to die right there."

Barbara, aghast at this breach of common sense, said. "Jason, what are you doing here? Are you crazy?"

A few minutes later, she received a phone call from the hospital. "They were frantic," she said. "Jason had never shown up for his radiation appointment. That's because he was with us at the time. I told the radiologist Jason was there at the hospital, visiting friends on another floor, and would be right down. I covered for him."

Then she turned to Jason and said, "I will harm you unless you get back to that hospital right now."

His cousins got him back to Manhattan, posthaste.

❦ ❦ ❦

Proud and independent as ever, Jason still wanted to skip treatment. "After the second operation, I tried to get him to do what he was supposed to do, to just show up there at the hospital and fight the cancer," Barbara said. "But I had to fight with him, just to get him to go along with the doctors. It was a constant battle." Team Vale once again went on special alert: watch out for this kid. "Come on now, Jason," Dr. Stephen Malamud, an oncologist at Beth Israel said. "No more shenanigans this time. You're going to get treatment." Jason had second thoughts, his resistance melting into reluctance.

"I prayed to God for guidance and wisdom," he said. "And He told me to get the therapy."

From December 1987 to January 1988, Barbara drove him to Beth Israel for radiation therapy and chemo treatments (the latter consisting of injections of vincristine, adriamycin and cytoxin). In combining radiation with chemo at the same time, the doctors went all-out to prevent a third tumor.

With each session, Jason grew sicker and weaker, succumbing to the toxins introduced to his system. Chemo is often a crapshoot, the treatment as harrowing as cancer itself, maybe worse. Quickly he lost his appetite and lapsed into nausea and vomiting. He dropped 40 pounds, his weight plummeting from 181 to 141. His temperature periodically soared as high as 104 degrees. He would wake in the morning and discover that overnight, his hair had shed in clumps all over his pillow. If he ran his fingers over his scalp, more came out. With his hair so patchy, Jason asked his friend Mike Messina to bring him razor blades, and he shaved himself bald.

The treatments indeed took a heavy toll. "I saw how sick Jason was during chemo," Barbara said. "That's what made all this so hard for me. He had no appetite. The radiation had burned his esophagus so badly that he could not swallow his saliva. I had to come in with some chicken broth or cream of wheat and spoon-feed him. He could not go to the bathroom. Nothing was functioning right. Some people with cancer get a certain death look. I had seen it in my own father. And that's the look I saw in Jason. His eyes were sunken. He had no eyebrows, no eyelashes, no hair. He was skinny. His hands were emaciated. A death look. For awhile he just laid in his bed at home with a pillow against the window during the day to keep the room totally dark. His room was like a crypt."

She would go down to his room and say, "Jason, I'll let in some light."

"No, it's okay, Ma," he would say. "It's all right."

"Are you sure? It's so dark in here."

"I want to be in the dark. I need this. I like it. It's good. It strengthens me."

As he lay swaddled in the soothing shadows of his room, Jason daydreamed about getting back to handball. Not even chemo and radiation could stop him from imagining his return to the sport. I have to get back to those courts, he thought. I'm going to get back and play.

"I thought about handball all the time," he said. "That's all I thought about. I saw myself making certain shots—boom!—and being even better than before."

He told his friends about his impending comeback. "The second I get better," he would predict to a partner, "I'm going to beat your butt." Look, he wanted to say. It can be done. You *can* come back from the dead.

To rise anew, Jason prayed every day. He knelt beside his bed and prayed until he heard God speak to him. He read the Bible, too, and found peace in sayings and stories about healing. In Proverbs, he read, "The spirit of a man will sustain him when he is sick." And he took this idea to heart. He would get better; nothing was going to stop him.

"The Bible is the best therapy," Jason said. "It tells you exactly what to do to get healed.

Barbara kept Pastor Marvin Boyce, of the Free Gospel Church in Flushing, posted on his progress. From the pulpit, Pastor Boyce would pass along the latest news and implore his flock to pray for Jason. Almost everyone in the congregation had known Jason since he first attended church there as a baby, and now parishioners wanted a blow-by-blow account.

Shortly after the second chemo session, the pastor came up with the idea of a 24-hour prayer chain. Jason had bounced back more slowly from the second round than he had from the first, and his oncologist had to cut the drug dosages for safety. Slowly Jason slipped deeper into the twilight between promise and doom, the chemo enfeebling him, and Boyce hoped the prayer chain would make a difference.

In a prayer chain, everyone could take turns praying for his recovery. Friends. Family. Neighbors. All people had to do was commit to a schedule telling what time they would pray. At the end of services, parishioners would sign up for a half-hour slot any time of day or night for the coming month. If you might miss doing your duty because of a conflict, you called another member of the church to take over your half-hour. In this prayer chain, dozens of people, maybe 50 or more, would be praying for Jason, hour after hour, for 24 hours a day, day after day, week after week, each one silently submitting a bid for his health and survival.

Still, Jason declined rapidly. After his third chemo treatment, his white blood cell count sank to practically nothing, and he needed a blood transfusion. He developed a fever and went back to the hospital for IV antibiotics and another transfusion. He returned home, but the fever led to an infection and now he refused, adamantly, to go back to the hospital for any more chemo. Why did he have to get so sick before he could get well? He felt like a yo-yo, as if he were just being strung along, never knowing for sure what was what. Cosgrove warned Barbara that Jason would die unless he let the hospital take care of him.

Finally, barely able to walk, leaning on Barbara and Joe for support, Jason gave in and returned to Beth Israel for a final chemo session, at a much lower dosage than before. Meanwhile, the participants in the 24-hour prayer chain kept at it. Bernadette and Jimmy Rosario prayed, and so did Ed and Ester Eliason. The Bensbergs, the Francos, and the McKenzies put in a word, too. The Messinas, the Mackens, the Nuccitellis—all patched themselves through on a special hotline to the heavens, as if dialing a toll-free number: 1-800-CURE-JASON. Almost everyone at the church prayed, each congregant chipping in a half hour of hope, all day and all night, the voices harmonizing, soaring skyward. The most potent medicine, they believed, was not chemo or radiation, but faith.

❦ ❦ ❦

After chemo, Jason hung out in Northern Cue, a pool hall on Northern Boulevard in Flushing, and took up arm wrestling for the first time since high school. His father Joe had taught him the sport at the age of 10, and for years Jason would dabble in it, never more than casually interested. Before the cancer, he could pin almost any other guy in his class, including some of the biggest and strongest.

What he really wanted now was to play handball or street hockey. He even bought himself a pair of $200 roller skates. Hey, let's get down to it. Time to bust heads. But before he could make a move, Cosgrove told him to forget it. The boy had lost three ribs and a chunk of his lung and some vertebrae. Any forceful contact could easily hurt him. He had to face facts. The two surgeries, the chemo and radiation, the infections and transfusions, had siphoned away his strength and his stamina. He could hardly stand. He still walked with a wobble because his legs, for now, were gone. No more handstands in the driveway, and no more quick steps in pursuit of a handball shot, either, at least not now. He needed a sport that called for short spurts of exertion but no legs. Hence, arm wrestling.

Now, in the smoky half-light of Northern Cue, with his frame all but wasted and his head shaven bald, Jason would look at a guy from across a pool table and think, I can take him. Over and over he heard this refrain in his head. Old habits die hard. He still needed to go eyeball to eyeball, to measure himself against an opposing force.

Now, though, he would lock hands with an opponent and give it all he had, only to lose. Still, he kept going at it, because even losing was better than nothing, better than living strung out on Percocet, with tubes in your chest. Here, in this pool hall, Jason would start his rehab. Dim and quiet except for the hiss of flip-top soda cans opening and the clack of billiard balls, Northern Cue was an environment conducive to recovery. He felt as if he were underwater, the pool hall reminding him of his hospital room with the curtains pulled shut, of his room at home with the pillow stuffed against the windows to keep out the light. Here he would begin to reel himself back from the lip of the abyss.

"Arm wrestling took my mind off everything else," he said. "It was therapeutic. And for some reason, I took it seriously. I wanted to get really good at it."

He would even arm wrestle Shorty, of all people. His real name was Paul, but because he stood 6 feet, 7 inches, everyone naturally called him Shorty. Shorty beat everyone in the joint and Jason was no exception. Just wait, Jason thought. I'll show you. One day Jason went so far as to tell Shorty, "When I'm better, I'm going to beat you." Cool, Shorty thought. The kid had plenty of nerve and they took a shine to each other.

For months, Jason challenged everyone in Northern Cue to arm-wrestling bouts. He resumed normal eating and put on weight and slowly regained his strength. "I prayed God would make me one of the best arm wrestlers," he said. "I felt that if I became one of the best, I would pay it back to God and glorify His name." Within a year, Jason had defeated all the arm wrestlers in the place—except one. But one night he locked hands with Shorty and pulled him down, too.

By chance, Jason heard about an arm-wrestling tournament held every summer at the Queens Day Festival in Flushing Meadows Park. He never realized he could compete in front of a crowd and maybe collect some money or a trophy. He called the promoter of the event for a flier and application form. With the contest only two months away, Jason practiced arm wrestling at every opportunity. He built a table in his bedroom basement, complete with handgrip pegs and rubber elbow pads at both ends, and there simulated matches, pretending to push down and pull back. And every day he got down on his knees, at the side of his bed, to pray. *I can win it. I know I can win it.* He thought of a particularly relevant passage from Samuel: "He trains my hands for battle; my arms can bend a bow of bronze."

Now at age 21, and weighing in at a much-improved 165 pounds, Jason competed in the arm-wrestling tournament at the 1989 Queens Day Festival. He won the first match, but lost the second, getting plastered in a blink. "First time I ever lost like that," he said. Still in the running, though, he faced off against the arm-wrestling champion of all of Virginia. Jason could tell by his grip that the guy had more power than he. Grip is the single most reliable measure of overall body strength; a strong grip generally means one is strong. "I knew it would be a hard match for me," Jason said. "I just wanted some respect and to put a fear into the guy. I decided that if he was going to beat me, I would make the match last as long as possible."

Instantly his opponent wrenched him low, pushing his quivering right hand to within an inch of the table. In such a predicament, the arm wrestler being overpowered usually loses within 30 seconds. But Jason held his own for a full minute, then two minutes, praying all along. "I held and held until I had nothing left," he said. Then Jason let go of the peg with his left hand, a foul, and the match resumed, until he fouled again, disqualifying himself from the match. "But it's not as if I lost," he said. "I never let the guy actually beat me." Jason had made his point, and so in this, his first tournament, he came in fourth.

He plunged into the subculture of arm wrestling. It's a sport where guys start at the kitchen table and the high school cafeteria. From hanging out with experienced grapplers, he learned the moves and the lingo. Hey, you could go with a wrist curl or a shoulder roll, a crunch move or a drag hook. You could take a high grip with your thumb, then hawk low on a guy and put the hammer down. Gradually he picked up inside tips. He saw that some wrestlers wore special arm gloves, covering wrist to bicep, that kept the muscles warm during breaks between matches. He learned that the human hand is the most intricate, specialized precision tool in all of nature—levers and hinges wired into a network of bone, tissue, ligament and nerve—and that you generate the most power if you keep your hand within 12 to 15 inches of your chest. He learned that you never shake hands with your wrestling arm because it's your prized instrument (besides, you might rub off the resin you patted on to give your grip some extra traction).

Most arm wrestlers compete for fun or ego or both, and almost none earn a living off the sport. They wrestle in benefits and fund-raisers, underwritten by sponsors such as Budweiser to cover the cost of trophies. They compete no more than once a month, because an individual may lock horns for as many as seven or eight matches in a single tournament. They have to watch out for those inevitable micro-tears in the shoulder and forearm; occasionally a guy comes away with a fractured arm. Competitors stay local, scraping together a few bucks out of pocket to travel to major regional or national tournaments out of state, and prizes seldom run higher than $1,000 or $2,000. But the sport is growing fast. About 40 of the 50 states have an arm-wrestling association, complete with executive director. And the annual world championships now draw at least 23 countries. Further, arm wrestling will become an Olympic exhibition sport in 1996.

Jason pulled matches in sports bars and at Lions and Elks Clubs, and subscribed to *The Arm Bender*, a quarterly magazine. Then, in February 1991, he drove to Stamford, Connecticut, to the Sports Gallery Cafe, for a Yukon Jack Arm Wrestling

Championship. About 300 spectators turned out to catch 103 competitors in 11 weight divisions ranging from 121 pounds to 243. Jason, weighing a sliver under 160 pounds, came away the winner of the lightweight division, with a $200 first prize.

"His attitude from the start was: learn, learn, learn," Johnny DiDonna said. "Keep practicing. Gain experience. He knew he was strong and had incredible speed and strength in his wrists. But Jason also had faith in himself, faith in God. He always believed he was going to win. And every time he lost, he saw it as a set of stairs to climb. He would think, 'Okay, I lost, but some good has come out of it.'"

A month later, he entered the New York State finals and won all six matches in the tournament, capturing another first-place trophy. In September 1991, he returned to the Queens Day Festival for another stab at victory. Defending champion Joe Vanero had won his weight division in the event for eight years in a row and seemed virtually invincible. The previous year at the tournament, Vanero had slammed Jason down in about a second flat. Now a crowd of about 500 onlookers, including a Vale entourage of no fewer than two dozen family and friends, gathered to watch the confrontation.

"I wanted revenge," Jason said. In the match, first Jason slipped out, then Vanero followed suit, and then out came the straps that bind wrestlers together and they tried again, both tied in place. "My family and friends chanted my name and screamed," Jason said. "I had goose bumps." This time Jason brought Vanero down in a flash, taking first prize. From then on, the arm-wrestling community officially designated him Lightning Bolt.

Al Virelli has seen Jason compete in about 50 matches. An accomplished arm wrestler himself since 1975, the tall, thin Virelli promotes tournaments and also acts as a referee and trainer in the sport. "Jason Vale is very strong," Virelli said. "But the first year I watched him, I could tell he lacked table time—experience. Once, I saw him go up against Jimmy Fitzimmons, a former national champion. Right away, Jason popped him over. But he had trouble finishing him off. Fitzimmons then had time to think, Hey, I've stopped him. What should I do to get out of this? Hook him? Roll him out? Fitzimmons knew how to get out of a losing position. And after about a minute, Jason lost. If Jason had had the table time, he would have beaten him."

Early on, Virelli realized that Jason was different from the others. "He seemed very soft-spoken," Virelli recollected. "He would just go off by himself between matches and stand on the side by himself and pray. I've seen guys before a match who do high fives or bang heads against a door or come out wearing a collar and leash. But Jason stays quiet. Keeps to himself and concentrates."

"Funny," Virelli added. "I was never aware he had had cancer. He never mentioned it to me. I heard about it from Andrew 'The Cobra' Rhodes, a championship arm wrestler out of Muskegon, Michigan. Cobra once got to talking with him and Jason told him about his cancer and showed him the scar. Cobra says it's one hellacious scar."

Before matches, Jason always got himself plenty prayed-up. Sometimes, afterward, he knelt and genuflected. One time he took down a guy who had gone nine years without losing, and Jason felt so grateful that he collapsed onto his knees and said thank you to God and walked outside into a parking lot and started crying. "I wish I could explain that feeling I get in a match," he said. "I'm not exactly sure what it is. It's like a heat in the middle of my body. Something inside me cries just as I get to the table. I cry because I've survived cancer. Because I'm there."

While attending Queens College in 1991, Jason ranked as the top middleweight in New York State, number-two in New Jersey, Connecticut, and Maine. He powered ahead with his arm wrestling in 1992. Competing as a middleweight (170 to 190 pounds), he went to Albuquerque for the World Professional Arm-Wrestling Association (WPAA) Tournament. In one match, he faced the 1991 national champion, in front of 2,000 fans, his largest audience ever. The opponent brought his hand to within a hair of the padded table, but Jason inched back to dead even, the audience shrieking louder and louder. Can I do it? he thought. Yes. Yes, I can. I can hold out longer than he can. Finally, he lowered the boom and shot his fist exultantly into the air. According to the WPAA, Jason finished the year ranked second nationwide in the 176 to 185 pound weight class.

"How good can Jason Vale be?" Virelli said. "He can be world champion. No question in my mind. He can definitely be world champion and lead the sport forward. All he needs is a little more training and technique. He's like no other arm wrestler. One in a hundred thousand like him come along. He's perfect for arm wrestling, just perfect. He has natural ability. He's a good-looking kid. He carries himself like a gentleman. He's come back from cancer. And he's only 24 years old. What else does he need?"

Arm wrestling is all about leverage, just like prayer. Anything to get a good grip. Anything to get over the top.

❦ ❦ ❦

Five years passed since his last operation and the angel with the dirty face had already lived a lifetime. Lived through the pain and the Percocet, the CAT scans, the defiance of doctors, the escape from the hospital, the radiation and the chemotherapy, and massages and spoon-feedings from his mother. Nothing would get him down. Nothing and nobody. He had fought against cancer just as he had Frankie Santos and almost everyone else on the block. And through it all, he had prayed his guts out. Five long years without evidence of cancer was long enough to mean he was almost certainly cured. Healed. To celebrate, the Vale family held no party, popped no champagne. They prayed.

At last glance, Jason was majoring in psychology and maintaining a 3.3 grade-point average. He had organized a team called the New York City Arm Wrestlers, who open every training session with prayer. He had also established a home-improvement business with himself as president. As for Barbara and Joe, five years later they were still paying the balance on his medical bills.

Why has Jason Vale survived? Could prayer alone do the job? Had he simply prayed away all traces of the tumor, no thanks to more conventional modes of therapy? Or had he come through this ordeal by dint of his resolve, his spirit of defiance and rebellion? One by one, the witnesses to his recovery come forward to take the stand and offer expert testimony.

"The doctors told us nobody had ever survived that cancer," his aunt, Joyce Vedral, said. "His chances of staying alive were nil. The doctors cannot account for his survival. But I'll tell you this. Jason told me God was going to heal him. He never believed for one second in the possibility that he would die from cancer. And he was never afraid to ask questions or to doubt the validity of the treatments. He refused to let the medical team do whatever it wanted and he questioned everything. He never accepted anything at face value."

Close friend Johnny DiDonna said, "All the doctors thought it would be fatal. I read the report about Askin tumor: everyone who had it died within a year. You just put two and two together. When he got cancer, I think I was more scared than he was." But Jason lived. He believed God would heal him, and He did. If you have a desire to live, you will. It was his whole attitude. He always believed the cancer would pass and he would keep going.

No one stayed closer to Jason throughout his trial with cancer than his mother. "It's hard to speculate what would have happened if Jason had had the radiation and the chemo after the first operation," Barbara Vale said. "The treatment might have so weakened his body that when the cancer came back, he might have lacked the strength to fight it. Who knows? Some people have a special purpose, and I think Jason is really a special kid. My friends ask me how I managed it. I deserve no credit. I think of the story, 'Footprints.' It's about a man walking along the beach with the Lord. Across the sky flash scenes from his life. Always he sees two sets of footprints in the sand, one from him, one from the Lord. The last scene from his life shows him low and sad, and he sees only one set of footprints in the sand. He could not understand and he asked the Lord to explain. The Lord said, 'During your times of trial and suffering, when you see only one set of footprints, it was then that I carried you.'"

The last word here goes to Dr. John Cosgrove, now the acting chief of the Tumor Service at the Kings County Hospital Center and the State University Hospital in Brooklyn. His expert opinion as a physician carries significant weight. "We all felt Jason was special," he said. "Some patients are tough; you know they're going to do well. Jason was such a patient. You could tell from that look in his eyes and his attitude: He knew he was going to recover. As physicians, we have a sixth sense about something like that. Of course, I could have done without his flights from the hospital.

"But otherwise, he was very committed to getting better, no matter what kind of tumor he had and no matter what anybody said. I've never seen anything like it before or since. He's determined, as well-focused as any individual I've ever met in my life. I've always felt that athletes have a singular toughness and sense of commitment. And he refused to let the disease get him down. A lot of other people would have given up. But Jason had one goal—to get better—and that must have helped him recover.

"Jason Vale is an inspiration to me as a physician," Dr. Cosgrove said. "Anytime I'm up all night on call, I think about how this determined 18-year-old kid fought an awful malignancy and came through it, and nothing I go through seems tough in comparison. When I'm tired and discouraged at the hospital, I think of Jason. I would venture a guess that after five years without evidence of disease, he's cured. And I believe his survival is a miracle. Now, we have no scientific proof, and it's impossible to measure, but I have no doubt in my mind. It is a miracle."

Amen.

Chapter 9

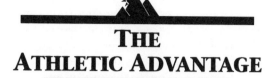

THE
ATHLETIC ADVANTAGE

Do top athletes possess an advantage over the average person in the struggle to cope with cancer? Are superior athletes endowed with a special, possibly unique attitude toward physical adversity— a Jock Factor, if you will—that promotes recovery from the disease? This chapter will explore those issues and get to the bottom line. It will present studies on both the cancer patient and the elite athlete—and trace the implicit connections between the two. It will look at the latest research on possible links between mind and body, and reveal the results of a survey, conducted exclusively for this book, on athletes and cancer. To wrap it up, widely recognized authorities on the respective psychologies of sports and cancer will venture opinions on the questions under discussion, leading to a consensus and, possibly, lessons for us all.

The first step in propelling the argument forward is a glance at the psychic dossier of the cancer patient.

❦ ❦ ❦

In the anatomy of cancer, the first insult to the psyche— and perhaps the most devastating—is the shock of diagnosis: *You have cancer.*

Patients wonder what kind of significance to assign to the crisis this news clearly constitutes. Studies show that because patients perceive cancer as synonymous with certain death, they respond to the initial diagnosis with pessimism, automatically assuming themselves to be terminal. Other reports reveal that as newly diagnosed patients look mortality in the mirror, they immediately tend to manifest such symptoms as tension, lethargy, headaches, anxiety, lowered self-esteem, depression, insomnia, uncertainty, reduced appetite, apprehension, sweating, and palpitations. They face confusion and conflict in trying to digest information and sort out emotions. Some refuse to believe or otherwise accept the diagnosis; others become angry with the physician who issues the verdict. The cancer eliminates a sense of structure in life, creating feelings of helplessness, loss of control, and social isolation. A nearly universal reaction to this diagnosis is fear—fear of the loss of work and relationships, fear of pain and disfigurement, fear of treatment, fear the disease will spread, fear of disability and death.

Patients at this stage face what appear to be umpteen decisions, major and minor alike. Which physician is best for me? Which hospital? Do I have enough life insurance? Will my spouse and I get to grow old together? Will I see my daughter graduate from high school?

Disturbing as it is, however, diagnosis is only the first in a series of ongoing challenges presented to cancer patients.

❦ ❦ ❦

During treatment, as a malignancy threatens to metastasize, the cancer patient typically encounters a series of woes. Biopsies, X-rays, blood tests, CAT scans, hospital stays, surgical procedures, chemotherapy, radiation therapy—all can take a traumatic toll. The disease disrupts even the smallest details of daily life and some patients withdraw and grow dependent to a childlike degree. Numerous studies show that treatment for cancer patients is often accompanied by increased anxiety, depression, anger, marital discord, occupational distress, sexual problems (including impotence, lack of interest, and sterility or infertility), despair, and a pervasive sense of helplessness and worthlessness in circumstances perceived to be beyond control.

In the case of chemotherapy—which always entails toxic exposure—patients are beset by a dread of injections, intravenous transfusions, and other medical procedures. Side effects of chemo range from mild to severe and are either temporary or permanent. Patients try to weather the wrenching mood swings, the emotional yo-yoing between desperate hope and profound despair. Radiation treatment, too, exacts a high price emotionally, as proved by a recent study. Researchers found that of 200 cancer patients, 124 reported themselves depressed before radiation treatment—and 199 felt depressed afterwards.

❦ ❦ ❦

Coping with cancer—what, exactly, does this phrase mean? Let's be clear. Coping is an effort, by thought or by deed, to manage, tolerate, minimize, and otherwise master the sometimes overwhelming physical and psychological demands of cancer. The most successful cancer patients—successful here meaning survival and return to some measure of normalcy—have discovered that the key is control. By either gaining important information, assuming a new perspective, or taking direct action, these patients restore a sorely needed sense of control over themselves, all in the belief that some semblance of control can affect the course of cancer treatment and perhaps even its outcome.

For example, a vital tool for coping psychologically with cancer is knowledge—knowledge of the disease and its treatment. Patients increasingly educate themselves about the disease, tapping the resources available to learn about the options for self-care, to exert control over themselves. The latest research suggests that such knowledge can ease fears of disability and death.

Studies have found that adopting a certain attitude may be a potent means of acting against cancer. To deal with the rigors of chemotherapy and radiation, patients learn to perceive the disease differently and to practice relaxation techniques, such as positive thinking, thought control, constructive self-talk, biofeedback, stress management, and music therapy. As they shift focus from the past to the present and the future, patients going through rehabilitation recognize the value of living a life of independence and self-determination. The evidence of success in these techniques is more than hearsay. Several studies report that before and during chemotherapy injections, progressive muscle relaxation, guided imagery, and hypnosis reduced nausea and vomiting, as well as anxiety and depression.

Of course, no one comes through cancer alone. Individual or group therapy enables patients to deal with the passages of the disease. A cancer patient often feels duty-bound to express his innermost concerns about the disease that has invaded his system—intimate confidences that may create a sense of community among other patients and, ultimately, a feeling of personal catharsis. A 1990 study at Stanford University underscored the value of such counseling sessions. Psychiatrist Dr. David Spiegel found that women with advanced breast cancer who attended weekly support groups for therapy sessions lived twice as long— an average of 18 months longer—as other women with equivalent illness and medication.

To cope well with cancer, patients are advised to live as normally and productively as possible and to participate in activities that recapture control, such as yoga, dancing lessons, karate, meditation classes. Cancer patients are schooled in banning negative thoughts and encouraged to confide in family and friends, freely expressing hopes and fears. As treatment continues, patients who follow this advice will realize they can look forward to many more good days than bad and can still expect to see more sunrises and sunsets.

Victor Frankl, a concentration camp survivor who wrote memorably about his suffering under Nazi oppression, knows something about coping strategies that can benefit cancer patients. While enduring the horrors of the Holocaust, he created a sense of meaning, order, and control in his mind, holding true to his personal beliefs and private reality to create a sense of predictability amid the random madness. Again, to adapt to extreme stress, it is a matter of employing the mind as an instrument of control. Studies have found that human subjects who believed they had control over the administration of an electrical shock showed fewer psychological responses to the jolt of voltage. What matters then, is not so much the objective reality—the chilling prospect of chemo or of death—as the perception of personal control.

Indeed, denial of the reality can be effective against cancer unless the refusal to face facts is prolonged or otherwise interferes with treatment or function. Studies show that cancer patients who demonstrate either denial or a combative spirit at the time of diagnosis, for example, have higher five-year survival rates than those who relinquished control through stoic acceptance and feelings of helplessness and hopelessness.

Psychologists who study cancer patients have formed a theory about a mode of survival called "self-efficacy." The idea behind "self-efficacy"—the process of making oneself effective—is that what you believe about your ability to perform effectively against cancer plays a prominent role in influencing how you think, act, and feel toward the disease. What a cancer patient believes about his levels of fortitude against discomfort and dread may deliver him a smoother passage through this crucible.

❦ ❦ ❦

Few better examples of self-efficacy exist among athletes who survived cancer than Jeff Blatnick. In 1982, the day before his 25th birthday, the big, burly Blatnick felt a suspect twinge in his neck. Oncologist Dr. Stewart Silvers detected a lymph node in his neck and diagnosed Hodgkin's disease. Surgeons soon performed a splenectomy, removal of the spleen, on Blatnick as a standard precaution because Hodgkin's often migrates to the spleen. Dr. Silvers also recommended daily radiation treatments for the wrestler, informing him that the five-year remission rate for such cancers, if observed early, is 90 percent to 95 percent.

"I was angry and scared," recalled Blatnick. "Everything came unglued for me during radiotherapy. The skin split on my neck. My shoulders turned red. My throat was so irritated that I had trouble swallowing."

By early 1983, however, the disease had apparently gone into remission. Nevertheless, Blatnick failed to make the U.S. National Wrestling Team that year. He says that the cancer and the accompanying therapy slowed his footwork, tightened his back, and numbed his fingers, leading to diminished strength, suppleness, and agility. Still, Blatnick persisted in training rigorously and eventually qualified as a super heavyweight in the 1984 Olympic trials. During the Los Angeles Olympiad, with millions of TV viewers aware of his struggle with cancer, the 6-foot, 2-inch and 248-pound Blatnick overcame one opponent after another. His comeback culminated in the final match, over Thomas Johansson of Sweden.

Before the event, his mother came over to say something about his deceased brother David, who had attended all his high school wrestling matches and encouraged his efforts. "Do it for Dave," she exhorted, and kissed him. After he won, 2–0, Blatnick, only the second American ever to garner a gold medal in Greco-Roman wrestling, exultantly dropped to his knees, crossed himself, and broke out crying. Sobbing still, he told a TV interviewer, "I'm one happy dude." About the message from his mother, he said, "It had a tremendous calming effect on me. I always dreamed I would do something for my brother."

Unfortunately, his jubilation was short-lived because a year later in a hotel room Blatnick felt a twinge in his upper right groin. He ran his fingers over the spot and felt a lump. A subsequent biopsy revealed a malignancy. Dr. Silvers told Blatnick that the cancer had recurred.

"I was mad and crying," Blatnick recalls about hearing the news. The next, most crucial step was chemotherapy, for six cycles of 28 days each. Despite such typical side effects as hair loss and nausea, Blatnick adopted the same attitude against cancer as he would toward a rival wrestler. "Some people feel embarrassed, humiliated, ashamed. But it's a process of survival. I refused to let the cancer rule me or intimidate me. I was ready to wear the stocking cap and take it on. Besides, who was I to think that my cancer would go away just because I'm an Olympic champion?"

Today a public relations consultant, motivational speaker, and occasional ESPN commentator, Blatnick grips cancer in a hammerlock. On July 22, 1992, he declared himself to be in remission, the absence of clinical evidence of disease after more than five years suggesting the likelihood of normal longevity. "As far as I'm concerned," Blatnick said, "I'm cured."

As for how he accounts for his survival, Blatnick said, "I never gave up."

But why not?

"Because I love wrestling. Because I was in charge. Because I took people who looked like Charles Atlas and wrapped them up in a knot."

Blatnick gives unstintingly of himself to the American Cancer Society and the Leukemia Society of America. "I have debts to pay," he explained. "I'm alive and others aren't. Talking with these other patients was a stronger medicine than any doctor gave me." In his public speaking engagements, Blatnick emphasizes positive thinking, easing fears about cancer. "Engulf yourself in life," he said. "Create a busy environment for yourself. This is not always an almighty whack to the back of the head. It's something you can work through. You can determine your own ends by the attitude you take. I'm a firm believer in faith. If you can accept making a sacrifice, you can still reach your goals."

❦ ❦ ❦

Now for a probe into the mental portfolio of the elite athlete.

William P. Morgan, Ph.D., a renowned sports psychologist, professor at the University of Wisconsin at Madison, and former advisor to several U.S. national and Olympic teams, began in the 1970s to apply standard psychological tests to athletes to see whether the results would enable him to predict how they would perform. In his search for an accurate yardstick, Morgan experimented with a slew of tests, including the Minnesota Multiphasic Personality Inventory, the Eysenck Personality Inventory, the Somatic Perception Questionnaire, the Depression Adjective Checklist, and the State-Trait Anxiety Inventory. Soon Morgan discovered that the most reliable measurement—the test most likely to forecast athletic success was the Profile of Mood States, now widely known among sports psychologists simply as "POMS" for short. POMS consists of a list of 65 words or phrases that describe moods or feelings (unhappy, tense, carefree, energetic, listless, grouchy, cheerful, nervous, unable to concentrate). Individuals are asked to indicate how well or poorly each word or phrase describes "how you have felt during the past week, including today." Respondents must then check one of five possible choices for each word: not at all, a little, moderately, quite a bit, or extremely. The resulting scores on a POMS test constitute a "mood profile" composed of combined scores in six general categories: tension, depression, anger, vigor, fatigue, and confusion.

Professor Morgan tried something new: he administered POMS to hundreds of superior athletes of college age, including marathoners, milers, and oarsmen. Result: athletes ranked well above average in vigor, with less tension, depression, confusion, and fatigue than non-athletes. "One general finding has consistently emerged," Morgan concluded. "Successful athletes in all sports possess superior mental and emotional health. They consistently show fewer signs of psychopathology and lower levels of anxiety, neuroticism, and depression than less-successful athletes and the general population." With POMS as his guide, Morgan accurately predicted nine of the 10 contenders who made 1972 United States Olympic wrestling team.

Earlier still, back in 1962, sports psychologists Bruce Ogilvie, Ph.D., and Thomas Tutko, Ph.D.—who have published numerous books, articles, and papers and delivered many presentations at clinics and seminars—founded the Institute of Athletic Motivation in California and developed a test called the Athletic Motivation Inventory, or AMI. The psychologists wanted to find out why some athletes succeeded more often than others, surmising that mental attitudes mattered as much as, if not more than, physical differences in athletic performance. Pioneers in the infant discipline of sports psychology, they hypothesized that elite athletes consistently achieved peak performance more because of an advanced mental state than the mastery of technical skills.

The AMI test consists of 190 questions. The answers—"true," "false," or "in between"—are designed primarily to measure motivation via characteristics that typically stand out in every successful competitive athlete. Drive—the desire to improve, compete, excel. Aggressiveness—asserting oneself, establishing presence, taking charge, forcing the action, making something happen rather than waiting for it to happen. Determination—the refusal to quit or accept defeat, the persistence to try and try again, the willingness to practice long and hard in a relentless quest to improve and win. Responsibility—holding oneself totally accountable for personal actions, recognizing mistakes and the need to change and improve, admitting errors and seldom making excuses or blaming others. Self-confidence—acting decisively, handling unexpected situations, never doubting the ability to meet challenges. Emotional control—handling pressures, staying cool, adjusting quickly, never getting upset by bad breaks or bad calls, delivering top performance regardless of circumstances. Mental toughness—accepting stern criticism and rigorous training from a demanding coach, recovering quickly from setbacks, seldom falling apart when the going gets tough.

More than 2,000 organizations, from high schools and colleges to Olympic teams and the pros, have applied this inventory of the psyche since 1963. The Institute of Athletic Motivation has conducted these psychological profiles on thousands of athletes in Major League Baseball, the National Football League, the National Basketball Association, and the National Hockey League, among other athletic organizations, to determine potential prospects. Conclusion? "Athletes are different from non-athletes," said William Winslow, current president of the institute. "Any athlete who has reached the top of his sport possesses certain mental characteristics in spades, or else he never would have gotten to the top in the first place. He's disciplined, he's energetic, he has the ambition to succeed, and he can endure discomfort and hardship with a thick skin. As a first-rate athlete, he's proved himself to be capable of overcoming adversity."

A study conducted at San Jose State University backed up these observations. Called "Personality Differences Among Athletes and Non-athletes," the research report applied the AMI test to specify any explicit disparities between the two groups. The study concluded that athletes consistently score significantly higher than non-athletes on such characteristics as "drive," "determination," "mental toughness," and "self-confidence." Similar studies, performed with the AMI at Northwest Missouri State University and the California School of Professional Psychology at San Francisco, confirmed the validity of these results.

As the illustrious psychiatrist Dr. Karl Menninger of the Menninger Clinic once put it, "There is considerable scientific evidence that the healthy personality is one who not only plays but who takes his play seriously."

The question is, Can athletes apply these qualities to a bout with cancer? Do such traits translate from sports to disease?

❦ ❦ ❦

Diana Golden fits this classic profile of an exemplary athlete as well as anyone—she possesses all the characteristics listed earlier, and then some. Skiing down slopes around the globe, Golden rated as one of the best skiers ever to come out of the United States. She garnered 19 national titles and 10 world championships. And she achieved such honors by competing in a style dramatically different from most skiers.

Golden hurtled along at 60 miles an hour, swerving precariously around mountainside gates, all on one leg.

One day in 1972, her right leg had buckled and the 12-year-old girl had fallen. A skier since age five, the New Hampshire native was diagnosed with bone cancer. Six weeks later, because such cancers more often than not prove fatal, her doctor delivered the inevitable verdict: a surgeon would have to amputate the leg. When told she would lose her leg to a point just above the knee, Golden said to the doctor, "Okay, can I still ski?"

A week after the operation, Golden stood one-legged for the first time, supported in part by a metal pylon with a prosthetic foot. She decided, out of curiosity, to remove the prosthesis. With shock she fully realized that nothing remained under her right thigh except air. "I cried all night," she recalled.

She learned to walk again, and seven months later—less than halfway through chemotherapy—she resumed skiing in the Cannon Mountains of New England, operating as a "three-tracker," gliding along on one ski and two outriggers. "I'd always skied, and I intended to keep on skiing," Golden said. "There was never any question in my mind about that. I thought to myself: All right, it's a leg and it's gone. It's not going to come back, so why waste my energy wishing for it to?"

"My parents never made me feel I had more to prove than anyone else," she said. When she was 16, her father said, "Do you think I care whether you win or lose? Well, I do. If you win, I'll be so proud, I'll tell everyone. But if you lose, it'll make no difference. I'll still love you."

And so, perhaps uniquely, Diana Golden became a topflight athlete *after* her brush with cancer. To train, she jogged and hopped through wind sprints—on crutches—up and down stadium bleachers. She jumped rope, lifted weights, played tennis, swam, did rock climbing, and practiced karate. She graduated from Dartmouth University, an English major, and applied her already well-formed athletic profile to the challenge of disability and came out a competitor.

"I never think about recurrence," Golden said. "If cancer comes again, I know now that I can deal with it."

She pioneered the idea, in U.S. Ski Association events, that disabled skiers should be able to compete against non-handicapped skiers—and was skillful enough to do so, often successfully. "When you're skiing hot, nothing else in the world exists," she said. "You never notice spectators on the sidelines, only the gates on the slalom course. You're not thinking about technique. You're ready to go beyond what you've ever done before. I'll think, Nothing is going to stop me from making the finish line. Once, in a race a few years ago, I heard a voice urging me on. 'Come on, Diane. Push it. Drive. Drive.' I thought it was someone else. But then I realized it was me."

The top female competitor on the U.S. Disabled Ski Team, she achieved the ultimate distinction at the 1988 Calgary Olympics. She competed in the giant slalom in Disabled Alpine Skiing and came away with a gold medal. The United States Olympic Committee bypassed all her two-legged competitors and named her Female Skier of the Year.

In 1990, Golden sought to reinforce her already fierce sense of independence. She headed to the Grand Gulch desert of southeastern Utah, where she camped out amid the sandstone, brush, and lizards. Alone. For five days.

"I get upset by the term 'victim' of cancer," said the cheery-voiced 29-year-old, who retired in 1991 and now speaks to disabled children at schools and camps and raises funds for cancer. "Victims of cancer are those who are no longer here. I'm not a victim of cancer. I'm still here. Cancer took away very little from me. I lost only a leg, not my life. When I skied, I never thought about whether I had one leg or two. But then, I was lucky. At a very young age, I saw other kids with cancer who failed to make it through. It's fair to say cancer changed my life radically. It motivated me to find a strength inside myself and become a world championship racer. It was almost a gift—all these possibilities came about that never would have happened otherwise."

❦ ❦ ❦

Does mental health affect physical illness? More to the point, can such intangible factors as attitude have a bearing on cancer, possibly as a benefit toward recovery?

Growing evidence strongly suggests an inextricable link between physical health and emotions or attitudes. Recent studies advance the idea that emotional states can change the course of a disease— that positive emotions, for example, may bolster immunity while negative ones depress it. Researchers studying the connection between the mind and bodily susceptibility to disease—a popular new field called psychoneuroimmunology—have found that neurotransmitters, immune cells, and hormones all act as messengers between our immune defenses and our thoughts and emotions. Accordingly, doctors around the country now routinely teach patients relaxation techniques as well as other alternative therapies such as biofeedback. The American Society of Clinical Hypnosis reports that more than 5,000 physicians use hypnotherapy.

Psychiatrists with expertise in psychosomatic medicine increasingly put forth the premise that the mind is a potentially powerful therapeutic instrument against diseases such as cancer. Indeed, a new breed of medical professional called a "psycho-oncologist"—with training in psychiatry and oncology—is emerging. Some preliminary clinical trials even indicate that stress may actually accelerate the progress of cancer.

William James anticipated such developments in his classic treatise, "The Varieties of Religious Experience," published in 1890. In this book, the philosopher discussed his concept of "healthy-mindedness" and referred to "a temperament organically weighted on the side of cheer and fatally forbidden to linger, as those of opposite temperament linger, over the darker aspects of the universe." In an apparent allusion to the virtues of denial, James described "the human instinct for happiness, bent on self-protection by ignoring." He added, "We divert our attention from disease and death as much as we can" and noted "the conquering efficacy of courage, hope and trust, and a correlative contempt for doubt, fear, worry and all nervously precautionary states of mind."

Norman Cousins brought such ideas into the mainstream in his landmark book, *Anatomy Of An Illness*. In his next book *The Healing Heart*, Cousins elaborated on these themes. He wrote, "The wise physician will encourage feelings of hopefulness and confidence for the same reason that he himself prescribes chemotherapy, radiation, or surgery... he does everything possible to encourage the patient to mobilize a strong will to live and all the positive forces that go with it... Increasingly, oncologists believe that the ability of a patient to express the full range of positive emotions—confidence, will to live, hope, love, purpose, joyousness—could have a significant bearing on the outcome... People sometimes discover within themselves capacities they never knew existed... Physicians have always believed in the usefulness and, indeed, the necessity of attitudes as aids in the healing process... And, since the human body tends to move in the direction of its expectations—plus or minus—it is important to know that attitudes of confidence and determination are no less a part of the treatment program than medical science and technology... Positive emotions can block the panic, foreboding, and depression that do such damage, inviting illness or intensifying it... The positive emotions, therefore, serve a specific and definite purpose in protecting the human body both in illness and in health... Serious illness should not be regarded as a pronouncement of doom but as a challenge, an adventure."

🐿 🐿 🐿

Next to death, cancer patients fear nothing more than pain. More than half of all patients with life-threatening cancers will at some point suffer pain requiring narcotics. Most of the pain associated with cancer is caused by growth of the primary tumor, but metastases, inflammation, and intensive treatments such as surgery, chemotherapy, or radiation can also bring on crippling pain. The pain involved in cancer is usually a series of discomforts and agonies, each prompted by a separate, specific cause, each needing a different diagnosis. At its most severe, the pain leads to anguish, disability, and a mortifying dread of death. Cancer patients take to a wide range of approaches, from narcotic drugs and biofeedback to hypnosis and relaxation training, to ease anxiety, promote a sense of control, and eliminate feelings of despair and desperation.

To the athlete, pain is a common denominator, a faithful companion, a given. Athletes virtually volunteer for a life of it, and blessed few escape its clutches. Pain—the word is derived from the Greek *poine* and the Latin *poena*, meaning payment or penalty—is a bill, payable on receipt, or, alternatively, a check the body hopes to bounce.

Few traditions in sports are as hallowed as that of the athlete who competes despite profound pain. In the folklore of sports, pain is the clay by which fans can mold an athlete into a hero for the ages. Think of Joe Namath hobbling to the line of scrimmage, of Micky Mantle with his scarred, buckling knees mummified in tape, of Muhammad Ali sustaining a fractured jaw in the first round of a heavyweight title defense against Ken Norton, then hanging on for 12 rounds to win by a decision. Think, too, of Los Angeles Dodger Kirk Gibson, gimpy but game, stepping to the plate in the first game of the 1988 World Series, in the bottom of the ninth inning, with his team down by two runs, with two outs and two men on base, and stroking a game-winning home run that barely cleared the wall.

Playing hurt is a matter of pride for most athletes, a byproduct of a Superman Syndrome. To the athlete, whose sense of identity is largely derived from his athletic prowess, the presence of pain sows doubts that he is physically invincible. The emotions evoked by pain—the dread and anguish—are often more of a challenge to an athlete than the physical fact of it. Pain is a smack in the face of ego.

The unwritten, unspoken credo: an athlete almost always plays hurt. With his flesh determinedly uncowed, the athlete may instinctively feel that his pain is an emblem of heroism. Bloodied and broken but unbowed, the athlete insists to himself that he nevertheless get out there, the embodiment of a bloodlust that harks back to the clash of Roman gladiators in the Coliseum. An athlete—not to mention his public, the team owner, the general manager, the head coach, and diehard fans—perceives his pain as an index of commitment, a barometer of character and courage.

For an athlete to confess to pain is all but taboo in the athletic community. As Sparky Anderson once put it, "Pain don't hurt." The basic code of conduct in sports militates against an athlete accepting, much less acknowledging or admitting to, the existence of pain. The hidebound macho ethic dictates that athletes keep a stiff upper lip, suffer in silence, and remember that real athletes feel no pain. "Elite athletes seldom complain about pain," said Boston sports psychologist Harvey Dulberg, Ph.D. "Athletes actually feel that they get points for playing in pain. If you ask an athlete if pain is bothering him, he'll most likely say, 'No, I never think about it, I ignore it, I know it'll go away. I'll ice it, it'll be okay.' They'll do whatever they can to make light of it, as if it's no big deal. It's not perceived as okay to talk about pain. They feel, If I can walk, I can play. It'll be for the good of the team. It's my job and I'm damn well going to do it."

According to Dulberg, athletes adapt to pain with an array of psychological defenses. Athletes may deny its presence ("Pain? Who, me? What pain?"), distort it to minimize its impact ("It's nothing serious, just a twinge; it'll go away soon enough"), and delude themselves about it ("It's only a minor concussion; I'll sleep it off and be ready tomorrow to play full-tilt").

Pain represents a classic mind-body showdown. Differences in personality may account for variable responses to pain and explain why some people are innately predisposed to heed its cues more vigilantly. Recent studies have shown that stable, contented, optimistic people demonstrate, on the whole, a higher pain threshold and tolerance than those who are by nature moody, negative, and pessimistic. Psychologists also believe that the attitude one takes toward pain can either aggravate it or, like a placebo, alleviate it. Personal expectations about pain are strongly influential: If we think we will hurt, we probably will—if not, not.

Athletes may find that a cheering crowd—or otherwise supportive fans and teammates, and doctors, and nurses in the hospital—can, in effect, drown out the voice of pain. What may count about pain, then, is context. Performing for high stakes, whether a Super Bowl ring or basic survival, can create an otherwise unattainable tolerance of pain. "Out in the thick of competition, when his reputation is on the line, even if the athlete should be in agony, he might not feel the pain at all," said Dr. Colin Stokol, director of the pain management program at Centinela Hospital Medical Center in Inglewood, California. "This need to perform pushes the athlete beyond the call of duty. He overrides the biological alarm for pain by force of will."

A study on pain at the University of Richmond in Virginia, led by psychologist Matt E. Jaremko, compared female basketball, field hockey, and track participants with female non-athletes. Conclusion: "Athletes in general have higher pain tolerance and thresholds." As Dr. Robert Kerlan, renowned sports orthopedist at the Kerlan-Jobe Clinic in California, has observed, "The pain threshold is unusually high among superstar athletes."

Attitude may be a potent analgesic in the athletic armamentarium, a will to win and the championship spirit enabling athletes to anesthetize themselves against pain. "A world-class athlete is a highly motivated, other-directed individual," Dr. Stokol said. "He will not let pain stop him. What separates him from others is the belief in his own physical superiority, in his healing powers despite pain, and in the idea that, no matter what, he will rise to play again."

Does this resistance to the pain incurred in organized sports carry over to the clash between an athlete and cancer?

❧ ❧ ❧

Among all athletes stricken with cancer, few have paid the price of pain more dearly than Dave Dravecky. Dravecky, starting pitcher for the San Francisco Giants, noticed a lump in September 1987—a desmoid tumor, also known as a low-grade fibrosarcoma—in the deltoid muscle of his pitching arm, near his left shoulder. "Running my hand along my left arm, I found a firm round shape under the skin on the upper arm, about the size of a quarter," he said.

In late 1988, orthopedic surgeon Dr. George Muschler of the Cleveland Clinic performed an eight-hour cryosurgery on Dravecky to remove the tumor. The freezing technique entailed in this procedure, as expected, killed 20 percent of the bone surrounding the tumor, rendering the humerus—the long bone in his arm extending from shoulder to elbow—even more brittle and vulnerable to fracture than before. The inevitable surgical scars prompted San Francisco teammate Kevin Mitchell to remark that his arm "looked like Jaws took a bite out of it."

The odds of such tumors recurring are about 50 percent; if they do, 90 percent come back within two years. Dr. Muschler told Dravecky that he would probably never throw again, much less pitch in the major leagues. "We presented the options to him," Muschler recalled. "Not to go back to baseball was the safest choice. But he's a man of tremendous courage and resilience." The pitcher knew that if he returned to the mound within two years of surgery, he risked breaking his arm.

"Dr. Muschler said that losing half my deltoid muscle would take away one of the three most powerful muscles in my arm," Dravecky said. "His greatest hope was that after intensive therapy, I would regain a normal range of motion and be able to play catch with my son in the backyard. I told him that if I never played pro ball again, I knew that God had someplace else he wanted me. I also said I believed in a God who can do miracles. And that if He wanted me to pitch again, I would."

Determined to pitch again, Dravecky slogged through an intensive rehabilitation program. Besides training with weights, he radically changed his throwing style, compensating for weakness in his left arm by relying more heavily on his rotator cuff and other shoulder muscles—painfully so. "Two weeks after the operation, I was able to lift my arms straight over my head," Dravecky said. "Other motions were severely limited, though. My therapist started by moving my arm for me. About three weeks after getting my surgical stitches checked, I was able to reach behind me to my rear pants pocket, take out my wallet, and set it down on the counter. It was the move Dr. Muschler had said would take months of rehabilitation to gain."

"From then on," Dravecky continued, "I had to focus on getting back normal use of my arm, then rebuilding arm strength, then developing my throwing ability. It was grueling work. That led to biceps curls with a one-pound weight, then bench presses, lap pull-downs, seated rows. And when I finally threw a baseball with Larry Brown, the physical therapist for the Giants, his first words were, 'How are you doing that?' I told him that as far as I was concerned, this was all a miracle of God."

Dravecky started pitching batting practice at Candlestick Park in June 1988. "Just being able to throw from the mound to home plate was a thrill," he said. He went to the Phoenix Firebirds, in the minors, and hung in there for nine innings one game, winning, 3–2. While he gathered himself down in the bush leagues, his fastball slowly climbed back to more than 80 miles an hour.

On August 10, 1988, only 10 months after the cryosurgery, Dravecky took the mound at Candlestick Park against the Cincinnati Reds. The scoreboard flashed a heartfelt message from all 34,810 fans in attendance: WELCOME BACK DAVE. "The crowd gave me an incredible standing ovation," he said. "That had never happened to me before. My heart was racing 100 miles an hour. Being given another opportunity out on the mound was really the greatest joy of my career."

Dravecky pitched eight innings, walking only one, his fastball clocked at a respectable 85 miles an hour. He had a one-hit shutout going into the eighth inning, then hung a slider that ended up as a three-run homer. But he still won the game, 4–3.

Five days later, in an outing against Montreal, the storybook comeback came to a wrenching end for the 34-year-old Dravecky. As he reached back to fire a fastball in the sixth inning, he crumpled on the mound in agony, grunting and writhing in the dirt. In the middle of his pitching motion, the humerus of his left arm—as Dravecky knew all along might happen—had snapped. "It felt like I lost my arm," he said about the incident. "I heard a loud pop just before my release point. My immediate reaction was to grab my arm because I thought it had left my body."

Soon after the tumor recurred, in October 1989, Dravecky decided to retire. Two operations removed the remainder of the deltoid muscles in his left arm as well as sections of its triceps muscle. Later, Dravecky returned to the Cleveland Clinic on a saddening mission—for radiation treatments to save his left arm from possible amputation. He also received a relatively new mode of treatment against cancer; the procedure involved sewing thin catheter tubes containing pellets of radioactive iridium into the arm.

In March 1990, President George Bush presented Dravecky with an American Cancer Society Courage Award. A little more than a year later, doctors at Memorial-Sloan Kettering Cancer Center amputated his left arm and shoulder. Still, his unbending religious beliefs pulled him through the pain. As Dravecky wrote in his first autobiography, "With Jesus Christ I can face any adversity... Now I will be playing catch with my kids, just as my father did with me. Baseball ends where it began: with a father and son, throwing the ball around."

❦ ❦ ❦

Does exercise during treatment, as in the case of Dravecky, enable cancer patients to cope better with the disease, even recover more swiftly than they might otherwise? Might such workouts serve well as an adjunct to conventional treatment?

The average cancer patient limits his activities during therapy and struggles against a mounting lethargy. All too often, physicians advise rest, sometimes in bed, and too much inertia is always counterproductive. Ample research supports the value of exercise in rehabilitation programs for cardiac patients, yet oncology has traditionally sworn by physical therapy alone. Exercising the whole body remains a relatively new idea in the physical rehabilitation of cancer patients. Rare is the physician willing to apply this principle—this exercise Rx—to cancer.

Results from several studies suggest that aerobic exercise has considerable promise in promoting functional capacity and well-being. Research on college students and faculty found that vigorous physical activity lowers both anxiety and depression, improves general mood, and enables individuals to cope better with emotionally taxing situations. Dr. John Griest and his University of Wisconsin colleagues, for example, found that running helped develop a sense of competence and control that spilled over into the rest of life and was as effective in alleviating depression as psychotherapy.

Clearly, fitness leads to a favorable self-image and positive attitude. In a recent study, some breast cancer patients undergoing chemotherapy exercised with moderate intensity on a cycle ergometer three times a week for 10 to 12 weeks while others remained relatively inactive. According to the ubiquitous Profile of Mood States, the exercising patients showed more vigor and less tension, anxiety, fatigue, dejection, and depression than the non-exercisers. The more active patients also improved more in functional capacity and feelings of internal control than the nonactive.

Athletes with cancer, by virtue of occupation, would be decidedly more inclined to work out as strenuously as possible during treatment. Most do, and probably benefit accordingly.

❦ ❦ ❦

No athlete has ever returned from cancer rehabilitation faster and more smoothly than Mario Lemieux, the 6-foot, 4-inch and 215-pound captain of the Pittsburgh Penguins in the National Hockey League. Lemieux, 27, noticed a lump on his neck in mid-

1992, but gave it no extra thought. Six months later he noticed the lump had grown and immediately informed his team physician, Dr. Charles Burke of the Allegheny Medical Center in Pennsylvania. On January 6, 1993, a CAT-scan revealed an enlarged mass, and Dr. Burke recommended removal. Two days later, Dr. Steven Jones took out a one-by-two-centimeter lymph node from his neck.

Following a biopsy, Dr. Burke gave Lemieux the news—he had Hodgkin's disease, a form of cancer. Thanks to early detection, he had a 90 percent to 95 percent chance of survival. "We told him that what he has is, as far as we're concerned, very curable, very treatable, and should not affect his career or his life," Burke said. "Then we told him what he had. He took it very well."

Lemieux, a nine-year NHL veteran and certifiable standout, had led the league in scoring three of the previous five seasons. The French-Canadian had played in six all-star games and carried the Penguins to two straight Stanley Cup championships. The previous October, he had signed a seven-year, $42 million contract. As of January 10, 1993, largely because of Lemieux, the Penguins had posted a 29–11–4 record. After only 44 games, with half the season left, he led the league in scoring with 104 points, 39 goals, and 65 assists, and had an odds-on shot at eclipsing the single-season scoring record of 215 points set by none other than Wayne Gretzky.

The news of cancer struck Lemieux like a blindside check. "Any time you hear the word cancer, it's scary," he said. "When the doctors gave me the news, I could hardly drive home because of the tears. I was crying the whole day. That was certainly the toughest day of my life." Lemieux had to tell the news to his fiancée, Nathalie Asselin, then six months pregnant, whom he planned to marry in June. The hockey star needed an hour to pull himself together for this task.

Lemieux had frequently faced traumatic injuries in his career— a severely sprained knee, surgery for chronic back spasms, a broken left hand—and always bounced back. "Mario will deal with this as he has everything else," said Phil Borque, a former teammate. "He'll take it in stride." Said his agent, Tom Reich, "His fortitude is off the Richter Scale."

Lemieux would begin radiation within two weeks. He met with his teammates in Pittsburgh before a night game against the Boston Bruins and delivered a pep talk.

"I'll be fine," he said. "No problem."

The next day Lemieux told a press conference, "I've faced a lot of battles since I was really young, and I've always come out on top. I expect that will be the case with this disease. This is another mountain I'll have to climb. I'm a very positive person by nature, and I'll be back when I'm 100 percent cured. Hopefully, that will be in time for the playoffs, and I can help us win another Stanley Cup."

Lemieux rested for two weeks, then began radiation treatment. "Mario is a world-class athlete," his oncologist, Dr. Theodore Crandall of Allegheny General, pointed out. "He will feel less fatigue than the average patient." Indeed, 12 days into his therapy, Lemieux began practicing sporadically with his team.

At 7:30 a.m. on March 2, less than two months after diagnosis, Lemieux underwent his 22nd and last radiation treatment. A few hours later, he chartered a small jet, took a nap at his hotel, and entered the Philadelphia Spectrum around 5:00 p.m. for a night game against the contentious Flyers. Lemieux donned a black turtleneck shirt under his uniform jersey because the radiation therapy had irritated his skin. Then, at 7:30 p.m., before a sellout crowd of 17,380, the public address system announced the starting lineups for both teams.

With the mention of Lemieux—this barely 12 hours after completing therapy—the fans gave him a standing ovation that lasted 58 seconds, some holding up signs reading GET WELL, MARIO, and finally the hockey star acknowledged the cheers and whistles with a wave of his stick.

Lemieux returned to the ice with a flourish. In the second period, he skated to the left-wing circle and, with a deft flick of the wrist, slapped in his 40th goal of the season. Moments later, he passed off for his 66th assist. Afterwards, his face flushed and slick with sweat, he gulped soda from a paper cup. "It feels good to be playing hockey again," he said in the locker room. "Overall, it was a good start."

❧ ❧ ❧

WRS Publishing mailed a 12-question survey about athletes and cancer to 261 members of the American College of Sports Medicine. With more than 12,000 members internationally, the Indianapolis, Indiana-based organization is the oldest and largest sports-medicine and exercise-science association in the world. The rationale behind this unprecedented survey was to establish some degree of scientific credibility for the premise of this book. Of all those members of the group who responded to the survey—mostly physicians but also exercise physiologists, physical therapists and nutritionists—65 percent reported having either treated or otherwise dealt with athletes who had cancer.

A chart on page 243 reveals the results of this survey. For now, let's look at a few of the key questions.

"Are athletes better equipped, physically, than non-athletes to face the day-to-day demands of cancer?" An overwhelming majority of 89 percent said yes, while 2 percent answered maybe and only 9 percent no.

"Would superior physical fitness give an athlete an advantage in dealing with cancer? Treating it? In recovering from it?" Again, a preponderance of more than three-quarters—78 percent, to be exact—said yes, with 13 percent saying maybe and 9 percent no.

"Does the ability to withstand pain give an athlete an edge over non-athletes in confronting cancer?" A sizable majority again prevailed, with nearly two-thirds—64 percent—answering yes, 27 percent maybe and only 9 percent no.

"Are athletes better equipped, emotionally, than non-athletes to cope with the challenge of cancer? With diagnosis? Treatment? Recovery? The persistent threat of recurrence?" More than half— 61 percent—said yes, 17 percent maybe, 21 percent no.

"Does attitude—the sort of attitude forged in competitive athletics—play a role in how athletes deal with cancer?" Almost unanimously, 91 percent responded yes, 9 percent maybe, and none no.

"Do you believe athletes deal better than non-athletes with the anxiety, depression, and despair to which cancer patients are so susceptible?" Here, with the relevant emotional disturbances delineated, respondents balked somewhat about the Jock Factor, with a marked majority—though fewer than half (47 percent)— saying yes, more than a quarter (28 percent) answering maybe, and fully 25 percent saying no.

"Do athletes have more focus, discipline, will power, stamina for dealing with the anxiety, depression, and despair to which cancer patients are so susceptible?" With a list of positive attributes juxtaposed with that of emotional ills, the sports medicine specialists gave athletes a 2-to-1 margin, with 67 percent saying yes, 13 percent maybe, and 20 percent no.

"Do you believe remission or cure rates for cancer are higher for athletes than for non-athletes?" Though this appears to be a dead heat—38 percent said yes, 24 percent maybe, and 38 percent no—consider that nearly one in four respondents remained unsure, thus willing to allow for the possibility of higher cure rates.

On the whole, the findings of the WRS survey are consistent with data from widely administered psychological tests such as the Profile of Mood States and the Athletic Motivation Inventory.

Though hardly the last word on the subject, the WRS survey strongly suggests that the deck is stacked in favor of athletes.

According to comments from respondents in this survey, athletes possess superior strength and stamina, are better accustomed to dealing with injury and rehabilitation, and are more attuned to themselves physically, the result of intimate familiarity with gut-busting training regimens. As a direct consequence, athletes are better prepared to tolerate pain and discomfort, stretch the barriers of fatigue, and withstand the numerous traumas—from invasive diagnostic procedures and extended hospitalization to major surgery and cycles of chemotherapy and radiation—imposed by cancer and its treatment. Further, athletes are significantly more inclined to work out during therapy and recovery, which helps them to retain some measure of robust physical condition. Thus, when it comes to pure physicality, the athletic advantage is virtually a given. As some survey respondents commented, it's a matter of survival of the fittest.

But athletics—and, to a certain degree, cancer—resides in the cerebral cortex as well as in the cells, muscles, ligaments, and tendons. An exquisitely engineered athletic specimen goes virtually for naught without the emotional characteristics that spell champion. As research has shown—the Profiles of Mood States, the Athletic Inventory, and now the WRS survey of sports-medicine specialists—athletes often have intangible but nevertheless singular inner resources, such as powers of self-control, discipline, focus, drive, self-confidence, and motivation. Athletes are predisposed, either by aptitude or occupation, to perceive cancer as a gauntlet tossed down, the ultimate opponent, a potential sudden-death contest. This attitude rouses the warrior spirit to arms. According to our survey, such traits prepare athletes to cope better with the unavoidable indignities—the anxiety, apprehension, and dread— that attend the diagnosis and treatment of cancer.

❦ ❦ ❦

Make no mistake: prick an athlete who has cancer and he or she will most certainly bleed. Not every world-class athlete is a model of character and courage in the grip of the disease, heroically immune to either the morbid terror a diagnosis customarily evokes or the hardships of therapy. Even an outstanding athlete in his prime, such as running back Ernie Davis of the Cleveland Browns, can fall victim to cancer. More recently, LPGA golfer Heather Farr, recovering from a mastectomy due to breast cancer, returned to tournament competition, only to drop out again with a series of debilitating recurrences.

Some sports-medicine specialists are skeptical of, if not blatantly hostile to, the notion of an athletic advantage against cancer. "I cannot fathom how anybody could establish an answer to these issues," said K. Calvin Thomas, M.D., internist for the New York Jets football team for 25 years and for the New York Islanders hockey team for five, in response to the WRS survey. "Whether athletes are better equipped emotionally against cancer is not only unknown but also not subject to assessment. All these are great questions, which, at best, are subject to theoretical opinions."

"Being an athlete could either help or hurt against cancer," said William H. Redd, Ph.D., a research psychologist at Cornell University Medical Center in New York City and attending psychologist at Memorial Sloan-Kettering Cancer Center. "We could say that it has benefits because athletes are more competitive, more disciplined, more accustomed to winning and being strong and healthy. But we could also say that for a perfect specimen such as an athlete, cancer is more of a violation."

"Athletes are highly achievement-oriented, with very high control needs, and illness—especially one as threatening as cancer—imposes a severe feeling of loss of control," stated Henry D. Childs, M.D., president of Health Investment Associates in Maynard, Massachusetts. "How well that is coped with depends a great deal on the adaptive mechanisms of the individual. Some athletes are worse about the emotional pain of loss of control, fear of the unknown, prolonged prescription drug regimens, loss of function, lowered self-image, depression, and anxiety. The whole cancer scenario, especially the uncertainty and length of it, might be harder for a personality oriented toward immediate action."

Cancer might actually turn out to be more galling, more daunting, and more taxing for the athlete than the average person, some medical experts observed. The athlete stricken with cancer might feel so trapped by the irony of his predicament—the paradox that although he is a profoundly physical being, an uncontrolled growth of abnormal cells in the body he once mastered has begun, unjustly and systematically, to insult and betray his sense of vanity and hubris—that he faces trials more onerous than does the average person. By this logic, an elite athlete is so wedded to his precious identity as an athlete, so accustomed to his physical excellence and virtual infallibility, that in a face-off against cancer, he might simply feel overmatched—out-muscled—and succumb all the more readily to, and indeed suffer amplified versions of, the anger and angst, the shock and bewilderment, and general malaise that go hand in hand with the disease.

Morton Bard, Ph.D., is a clinical and social psychologist and a former vice president of the American Cancer Society. A pioneering researcher in the 1950s on the psycho-social effects of cancer, Bard studied "beliefs of significance" in cancer patients—what they thought brought on the illness—at Memorial Sloan-Kettering Cancer Center. He has counseled thousands of cancer patients over several decades.

"Athletes are the epitome of function and performance, with finely honed capacities," Bard said. "They are prototypically devoted to performance. If a person is organized internally, where the joy of function and the gratification yielded thereby are held in some kind of balance or harmony, then that individual is likely able to withstand adversity and overcome the disabling effects of a disease like cancer. Now, I think some athletes, in an encounter with cancer, probably get into a mastering mode— mastering cancer as they have other challenges. It brings out the pride in body, the competitive streak, the will to win. It might be based on some kind of narcissism. But other athletes might collapse under the weight of cancer, fall into a funk, and feel defeated by being unable to overcome what is seen as a serious defect. In cancer, the self is violated and function is disturbed and disordered. Tremendous adaptive demands are placed on the individual to make up for the rupture, the rending, of that self. It may be extraordinarily threatening for an athlete if something as out of control as cancer violates his mastery over his body. Some may see it as a challenge to overcome by sheer dint of will, but others will be floored by it.

"I have seen nothing in the form of evidence that would persuade me—and I can theorize and hypothesize as well as the next guy—that athletes are unique in this regard," Bard said. "Yes, athletes do have great concentration, but then that's also true for actors, scientists, and others who have to focus with intensity to perform at higher levels. It's not a question of occupation so much as how the individual person is constituted to deal with a life-threatening illness. That said, I believe athletes probably vary as widely in response to the insult of cancer as anyone else. I suspect that they are no different from other people."

❧ ❧ ❧

Clearly, opinion on the subject is divided.

William Winslow, president of the Institute of Athletic Motivation in Redwood, California, has pored over thousands of test scores on the Athletic Motivation Inventory. Winslow is unequivocal in his view that athletes do possess psychological traits conducive to waging a successful campaign against cancer. "A number of those characteristics enhance the probability of mental success against cancer," Winslow said. "In terms of treatment for cancer, an athlete has a proven endurance to persist against pain and suffering, and the self-confidence that's so valuable in confronting and overcoming a disease like cancer. An athlete is undoubtedly more competitive than anyone else, too— he wants to win at anything, especially if it's a life-threatening disease."

Bruce Ogilvie, Ph.D., a San Diego State University professor emeritus who co-developed the Athletic Motivation Inventory, is widely regarded as the dean of American sports psychology. Now past 70, white-haired and handsome, Ogilvie conducted pioneering research in the field in the 1950s and 1960s. He has served as a consultant to many elite athletes, including Olympic hopefuls and professionals in the National Basketball Association, the National Football League, and Major League Baseball.

"Elite athletes are more stable and tend to be more optimistic and tough-minded than non-athletes," said Ogilvie. "You can find statistic differences to that effect. When confronted with a tragedy or a disability or a diagnosis of cancer, they usually face reality directly and are able to maintain a stable, secure adapting style. They engage in mental healing strategies because they are self-determiners. An athlete, rather than let a crisis deflate him and rob him of the power to manipulate or change events, sees it as a problem to solve. The most successful cancer patients will engage in this kind of problem-solving rather than submitting to depression, the death knell for anyone with a diagnosis of the disease. Now, the suggestion is that these athletes are by nature better able to withstand stresses and have a hardiness, a capacity to bounce back, and see adversity, such as the threat of death from cancer, not as a statement of personal worth or a definition of inadequacy but, rather, as an opportunity to face a challenge."

Ogilvie, now retired in northern California, leaned back in his chair and spoke slowly now. "The sacrifice and commitment to become excellent in sport can have a carryover effect for a cancer patient," he said. "Frequent success in overcoming obstacles reinforces the belief in further success. Rather than retreat into the view of 'It's hopeless, there's nothing I can do,' athletes have a deep conviction that because they have succeeded in dealing with pain and injury, they can do something to actually inhibit the disease process itself."

A recent study of Jews who survived captivity or hiding during World War II furnishes a provocative parallel to the matter of athletes with cancer and a possible example of the carryover effect Ogilvie cited. According to Dr. William B. Helmreich, a professor of sociology and Judaic Studies at the City University of New York, some survivors of Nazi genocide achieved more personal and professional success than other American Jews of comparable age, with more stable marriages and less need to seek psychiatric help. Helmreich finds that the traits that enabled Jews to survive the Holocaust—a turn-on-a-dime adaptability to changing circumstances, a readiness to take the initiative, and a ferociously stubborn tenacity—may also account for later successes in life. "I found a widespread ability to think quickly, size up a situation, break down its complex elements, and make an intelligent decision," Dr. Helmreich said. He also noticed that Holocaust survivors had a distinct tendency to divorce themselves mentally from the pain, fatigue, anxiety, and depression typically brought on by the horrors of long-term captivity. The upshot is that these survivors applied personality traits developed of necessity under extreme duress toward success in future circumstances.

Harvey Dulberg, Ph.D., is a nationally recognized sports psychologist, a psychology lecturer at Boston College, and the author of a nationally syndicated newspaper column called "Sports Shrink." A former competitive tennis player in college, he has counseled athletes for more than 20 years, from professionals and aspiring Olympians to an 8-year-old whose anxiety before Little League contests routinely induced him to throw up.

"I believe that an athlete is in a position to deal better with cancer and even have a better chance of overcoming the illness than the average person," Dulberg said in his office in Brookline, Massachusetts. "I'd like to think that athletes would have higher remission rates than non-athletes, that a study would show athletes responding better to treatment and living longer. Those who are successful have certain personality traits—some inherent and biologically given, others learned—that they can call to the fore when needed to deal with the problems of a life-threatening illness.

"Having worked with many injured athletes, I'm comfortable speculating on this idea," Dulberg said. "I see these athletes with cancer as never taking no for an answer, really fighting with every ounce of strength to get back into shape, being very driven to reach a goal. They take a more active role in treatment than the average person: If a doctor tells an athlete what to do, he's more apt to do it. I think a world-class athlete, to overcome an illness like cancer, is going to have that cockiness rather than lay down and die.

"We're talking about redirecting energies, really—from athletic competition to disease. Resistance to pain on the field, for example, translates to the cancer patient. An athlete has learned to focus, to control his emotions, to put the rest of his life aside until the competition is over, in order to succeed consistently. That discipline turns out to be an invaluable asset against cancer, too. The competitive streak, the pride in physical accomplishment, never go away. The worse the outlook, the more they arouse themselves and say, 'I'll prove otherwise.' I believe that once an athlete, always an athlete, even in the hospital. Remember: The doctor told Dave Dravecky he might break his arm if he pitched again. Dravecky said, 'I'll take the risk.'"

The last word here goes to David Wellisch, Ph.D., a professor of medical psychology at the University of California at Los Angeles School of Medicine and a specialist in counseling cancer patients. Active with the American Cancer Society, Wellisch is affiliated with Vital Options, a free-standing Los Angeles center that offers counseling and coping strategies to cancer patients 18 to 40 years old—the same age range as most athletes profiled for this book. The psychologist—who, by the way, plays racquetball twice a week—has researched the psychology of cancer for more than 20 years. Cancer is a personal issue for Wellisch: his mother died from the disease in 1973, his father 10 years later, inspiring his intense interest in the mental dynamics of cancer. He took considerable time and care to ponder—and illuminate—the proposition about an athletic advantage.

"The athlete is well-organized and goal-oriented, perfect qualities for dealing with the pain, the fatigue, and the tremendous mental stresses of cancer," Wellisch said. "He has a capacity to focus and actualize, to build on his innate strengths to function better and achieve more by mobilizing his emotional resources— also differences that could add a great deal of an edge against cancer.

"To deal with either athletic competition or cancer calls for an extreme degree of self-reliance. A cancer patient, to get through treatment, has to have the same kind of mental set—the self-possession and self-absorption, the functional withdrawal into the self—as an athlete needs to compete successfully. We teach cancer patients self-hypnosis and relaxation exercises so they can withdraw into themselves and be very focused, to the exclusion of everything else. It's a process called introjection, by which you internalize your coach or doctor and now have a person inside you who gives you support and pep talks."

Wellisch paused to look out the window of his UCLA office for a moment.

"The whole idea for the athlete is to be in control of an event, of his body, of his mind," he said. "When you hone yourself for peak performance, you have to stay in control, to be single-minded, with a narrow, fixed focal point. That's what sports have trained him to do—to be self-sufficient, to focus, to depend on defense mechanisms to protect himself from pain, suffering, deprivation, anxieties, and other normal feelings, to maintain an even keel, to cut off the past and live in the present and the near future. With cancer, you have to determine whether you're going to control it or it's going to control you. The best form of coping against cancer—as opposed to the avoidance or escapist approach—involves confronting and attacking. Now here, too, is where I believe athletes are better prepared than the average person. The survival instinct in these people is so profound that they can push themselves through almost anything.

"An athlete deliberately limits his conscious experience," Wellisch continued. "It's like self-hypnosis, as if he'll anesthetize himself, distancing himself from the uncomfortable or anxiety-producing or noxious stimuli. An athlete with cancer will be able to go someplace else in his mind and close himself off from normal feelings of pain and discomfort. Athletes do this all the time, this limiting of conscious experience, this distancing from normal feelings, only because they have to.

"Athletes take what they learned on the field and apply it to cancer. They have a confidence born of previous experience in dealing with serious obstacles. They think, 'I've met difficult, seemingly hopeless circumstances before and gotten on top of it. I'll take care of this, too.' I believe a learning state is cross-applicable.

"Is an athlete likely to deal more effectively than a non-athlete with cancer from a psychological standpoint?" Wellisch pondered. "Yes, I believe that there is an advantage to being an athlete—a so-called Jock Factor. The successful athlete is different even from other successful individuals such as business executives because his stock in trade is the linking of psyche and soma, mind and body. The athlete knows from intimate experience all about how the mind and body are connected and can influence each other. I believe the profile of the successful athlete is the same as the profile of the successful cancer patient. Top athletes are survivors.

And that's exactly what it takes to be a successful cancer patient—
a survivor."

                            ❦ ❦ ❦

But hold on a second now. The ice here is not only slippery
but also thin. Some sports medicine specialists, reluctant to
hypothesize about this putative athletic advantage, say: Show us
the evidence. And, indeed, aside from human-interest narratives,
the literature on the topic of athletes with cancer is scant. Nobody
has yet conducted surveys, much less scrupulously randomized,
double-blind clinical trials, of athletes who survived the disease.
The data on this theme remain vastly more anecdotal than
empirical, more theoretical than conclusive. The authorities quoted
here have ventured opinions that are admittedly speculative and
extrapolative. And whether the remission rate for cancer, to take
just one aspect of the overall issue, is higher among athletes than
the average person remains wholly undocumented.

One can ill-afford to generalize about this subject and risk
misleading the general public with charlatan claims. So let's get a
few caveats and disclaimers on the table here. Competitive athletes
with cancer are usually younger than most cancer patients. As
such, they have relative youth as a weapon against the disease
and go largely untouched by the more fatal forms of cancer, such
as those attacking the lung and liver. The stage at which cancer is
detected also has to be taken into account. Most of the athletes in
this book are under 40 years old and had a form of cancer that
was uncovered early so that it posed little threat to life and limb.

Moreover, how well a given athlete responds to cancer—to the
dark omens conjured by the alarm of diagnosis, the tribulations
of treatment, the menace of recurrence—depends largely, if not
entirely, on whether he has proved equal to previous challenges
and crises. Cancer is cancer, an aberration of runaway cells, and
people are people, whether one swings a baseball bat for a living
or computes profit-and-loss statements. Sometimes, of course,
cancer just plain refuses to play by the rules, ungoverned by
either conventional or alternative medical therapies, beyond the
dictates of attitude, its malignancies multiplying exponentially,
the disease both mysterious and monstrous. Many a person who
never set foot on a basketball court is well-organized and goal-
oriented, his hatches battened down against the buffetings of
doubt and desolation, determined to succeed at all costs. Thus,
not every sedentary accountant with a tumor should, as a matter
of course, write himself off as terminal. Nor have athletes cornered

the market on exemplary coping skills, for either life in general or cancer in particular. An athlete is issued no guarantees that the force of will alone, however formidable, will form a force-field protection against emotional hardship, much less domesticate a disease.

❦ ❦ ❦

All the same, many authorities assert, and the research compiled indicates, that this theory that athletes have an advantage over the average person against cancer deserves, at the very least, serious contemplation. UCLA psychologist and cancer specialist David Wellisch proposes a study comparing, say, 25 athletes who have survived cancer with 25 non-athletes who have come through the disease, each group matched according to such factors as age, form of cancer, and ethnic heritage. Given the necessary funding, Wellisch would administer a standardized questionnaire on states of mind during diagnosis, treatment, and recovery to determine any differences between the groups. Though small-scale and less than definitive, this study could serve as a first step and encourage subsequent research.

We've also established, with some degree of certainty, that fitness and exercise are almost invariably beneficial to cancer patients. Physicians should therefore prescribe exercise for cancer patients more aggressively than is the case now, if only as a means of elevating overall mood. The intensity and duration of exercise would depend on the patient and the circumstances. But with precautions taken against undue pain, fatigue, or muscular stiffness, patients who start slowly on a customized exercise program and progress at a suitable pace may benefit accordingly. Said Wellisch, "Exercise promotes the belief that if you can walk a mile, you can take another round of chemo."

Exercise may not only deliver a therapeutic payoff for cancer patients but also—as recent studies of breast and colon cancer patients have suggested—may help prevent the disease as well. Keeping this exercise Rx in mind—and remembering that one in every three Americans now alive may someday contract cancer—the general public would have yet another major incentive to stay in shape.

❦ ❦ ❦

But in the end, the most persuasive evidence for a Jock Factor lies in the stories of athletes who have overcome cancer. So many athletes with the disease, including a few who were counted out and all but left for dead, have come through, offering compelling, albeit still preliminary, proof of the existence of an athletic advantage.

PGA golfer Gene Littler is yet another case in point. In 1972, he had amalignant melanoma on his left arm. Surgeons removed two muscles leading directly to nerves in his shoulder that governed his swing, leaving the arm hopelessly weak. Littler returned to the golf course five weeks later, his left arm still in a sling, to contemplate a comeback. Then, to rehabilitate himself, he tried swimming with one arm and almost drowned. Merely ten weeks after surgery, he played nine holes of golf for practice, and a month later he played in a tournament, scoring birdies on the last two holes and winning the event. Within a year of the operation, Littler captured no fewer than four major tournaments, including the prestigious Westchester Open. Arnold Palmer commented, "Gene has whipped cancer, and he's playing golf because it's his game and it's something he loves to do."

Take the example of Mike Gallego of Tacoma, Washington. In 1983 the 23-year-old baseball player was diagnosed with testicular cancer. Gallego underwent surgery and radiation, losing 15 pounds in the process, only to come back two years later as an infielder for the Oakland Athletics and, most recently, for the New York Yankees. Also in 1983, doctors discovered that an 18-year-old named Keith Kartz had tumors in his stomach and lymph nodes, but he returned to high school football practice only six months after surgery and chemo. Kartz ultimately parlayed this perseverance into a position as the starting center for the Denver Broncos in the 1987 and 1990 Super Bowls.

Consider, too, the cases of amateur competitors who struggled back against cancer, perhaps all the more impressive for the absence of money and fame as motives. Julie Gibson, a 34-year-old New York City textile saleswoman who ran seven miles a day, developed leukemia, but while in the hospital she persisted in powerwalking through the corridors for two hours a day, wearing a four-pound weight around each wrist and a two-pound weight around each ankle. Lee Modjeska, 59, a highly successful attorney and professor of law at Ohio State University, was diagnosed with a rare and aggressive thyroid cancer in 1987. The next year he took up Tae Kwon Do at the urging of Master Joon Pyo Choi, a former U.S. Olympic coach and Korean national champion. "The stronger you keep yourself mentally and physically," Choi told him, "the better you're going to do throughout this process." Modjeska studied the martial art for three-and-a-half years, earning a black belt.

Finally, the athletes whose trials against cancer are detailed in previous chapters voice the most eloquent testimony in favor of an athletic advantage. Witness 50-plus Connecticut attorney Barbara Norman, stricken with breast cancer, still mourning the death of her beloved husband, gagging from chemo, yet forcing herself, thanks to urging from training companion Kathy Salvo, to trudge a few miles on a muddy course in a slashing rain, then going on to nab third place in her age group in the vaunted Hawaiian Ironman Triathlon. Reflect on Welsh-born soccer star Clive Griffiths, vomiting through chemo for testicular cancer, wasting away into a husk of himself, then staggering into a hospital delivery room, white-faced and weak, to see his baby girl Meredith born—and then returning to captain his Kansas City Comets to the playoffs. Behold veteran marathoner Fred Lebow, given no more than six months to live with an inoperable brain tumor, drawing strength from all his brothers and sisters, renewing his faith in Judaism, hobbling along hospital roofs and corridors to keep fit, then coming back, at the age of 60, to totter through the very New York City Marathon he had created from scratch 20 years earlier on his kitchen table. Replay the images of Jason Vale, handball hotshot and neighborhood pugilist, who never once backed down from a bully, agonized by a rare growth in his chest that all his doctors believed would kill him, praying his guts out through two traumatizing operations, twice fleeing from the hospital to minister to himself on his own terms, then, after simultaneous chemo and radiation, transforming himself into an iron-willed arm-wrestling champion. Finally, think of a small-town Texas teenager named Jeff Banister, steeling his resolve through seven operations for a bone cancer threatening to devour his left leg, coming back to win a baseball scholarship, only to sustain a broken neck in a home-plate collision and lay in traction at risk of a lifetime sentence as a paraplegic, daydreaming during all his months imprisoned in the hospital of the sport he loved to play, then teaching himself to walk again, logging four years of hard time in the minors and, at long last, at the advanced age of 26, getting called up by the Pittsburgh Pirates and, in his only major-league game, in his only pro at-bat, legging out a pinch-hit single.

So: Yes. Yes, in all probability, the athlete will chalk up an edge over the average person in going against cancer. Yes, the athlete can program himself to limit his conscious experience under the most extreme duress, to deafen his ears to the strident voices of pain and fatigue and general distress. Yes, it's a question of survival of the fittest, a matter of cross-application—the channeling of energies previously directed into sports toward cancer instead. No, sport is not the same as cancer, but neither is it altogether different. Still, just as sports concentrate the mind wonderfully, so does the crisis of cancer.

The lesson here is that if we think like athletes, if we assume an athletic attitude, if we take just the right stance at the plate as the pitch we call daily life zooms toward us, we may give ourselves a leg up on any setback, including cancer. As Cornell University psychologist William H. Redd pointed out—and this bears remembering as a key to the Jock Factor—"What we do know for certain is that a history of good mental health is a reliable predictor of coping effectively with the distress of cancer."

All the athletes in this book share certain emotional qualities, characteristics that led not only to athletic excellence but also to the winning of a contest against cancer. Adaptability. A competitive drive. A single-minded focus. A preference for self-reliance. A refusal to feel singled out, persecuted, or scapegoated. An intense desire to return quickly to the sport of choice. A pragmatism that says, What is *is*, what happens *happens*. A realization that no one gets through cancer alone, but, rather, needs to trust in friends, family, teammates, and, optionally at least, God. An understanding that attitude is almost a muscle in itself, a muscle that should be routinely flexed and toned—that your bearing, your perspective on what's around you and inside you, has a hand in any quest to succeed, whether on the gridiron or in the radiation unit. An acknowledgment that just as athletic events are won move by move, point by point, cancer is endured test by test, treated drug by drug, destroyed cell by cell. And, above all else, no matter how trying the circumstances, a will to live; the instinct, the spirit, the courage to do whatever it takes to survive.

WRS SURVEY ON ATHLETES AND CANCER

1. Are athletes better equipped, physically, than non-athletes to face the day-to-day demands of cancer?

        yes 89%   **maybe 2%**   **no 9%**

2. Would superior physical fitness give an athlete an advantage in dealing with cancer? Treating it? In recovering from it?

        yes 78%   **maybe 13%**   **no 9%**

3. Are athletes better equipped, emotionally, than non-athletes to cope with the challenge of cancer? With diagnosis? Treatment? Recovery? The persistent threat of recurrence?

        yes 61%   **maybe 17%**   **no 21%**

4. Does the ability to withstand pain give an athlete an edge over non-athletes in confronting cancer? To endure fatigue?

        yes 64%   **maybe 27%**   **no 9%**

5. Does attitude—the sort of attitude forged in competitive athletics—play a role in how athletes deal with cancer? This is, might a competitive mind-set, a warrior mentality, have an advantage against cancer?

        yes 91%   **maybe 9%**   **no 0%**

6. Do you believe athletes would deal better than non-athletes with the anxiety, depression and despair to which cancer patients are so susceptible?

        yes 47%   **maybe 28%**   **no 25%**

7. Do athletes have more focus, discipline, will power, stamina for dealing with the anxiety, depression and despair to which cancer patients are so susceptible?

        yes 67%   **maybe 13%**   **no 20%**

8. Do athletes in general bring an advantageous and distinctive physical and psychological makeup to a confrontation with cancer?

        yes 80%   **maybe 13%**   **no 7%**

9. Is regular strenuous exercise a possible prophylactic measure against cancer? A legitimate form of therapy for cancer patients? Is an athletic lifestyle an aid in overcoming cancer?

        yes 50%   **maybe 26%**   **no 24%**
        yes 58%   **maybe 18%**   **no 24%**
        yes 62%   **maybe 24%**   **no 14%**

10. Have you ever treated or otherwise dealt with athletes who had cancer?

        yes 65%   **no 35%**

11. Do you believe remission rates or cure rates for cancer are higher for athletes than for non-athletes?

        yes 38%   **maybe 24%**   **no 38%**

12. David Wellisch, a professor of medical psychology at UCLA School of Medicine says, "The profile of the successful athlete is the same as that of the successful cancer patient... the athlete is well-organized and goal-oriented, perfect qualities for dealing with the pain, the fatigue and the tremendous mental stresses of cancer." Your reaction?

        agree 55%   **unsure 41%**   **disagree 4%**

*R*obert Brody has written about sports medicine and sports psychology for many publications, including *Esquire, GQ, Omni,* and *Sport* magazines An award-winning writer with a speciality in health issues, he is an avid recreational basketball and tennis player. He lives in Forest Hills, New York, with his wife, Elvira, and children, Michael and Caroline.

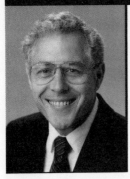
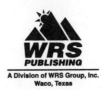